Essential Learning Skills for Health Professions Students

Khalid A. Bin Abdulrahman • Hassan Darami
Editors

Essential Learning Skills for Health Professions Students

Springer

Editors
Khalid A. Bin Abdulrahman
Department of Medical Education, College of Medicine, Imam Mohammad Ibn Saud Islamic University (IMSIU),
Riyadh, Saudi Arabia

Hassan Darami
Department of Obstetrics & Gynecology and Medical Education
College of Medicine,
Imam Mohammad Ibn Saud Islamic University (IMSIU)
Riyadh, Saudi Arabia

ISBN 978-981-96-5669-1 ISBN 978-981-96-5670-7 (eBook)
https://doi.org/10.1007/978-981-96-5670-7

This Springer imprint is published by the registered company Springer Nature Singapore Pte Ltd.
The registered company address is: 152 Beach Road, #21-01/04 Gateway East, Singapore 189721, Singapore

Preface

Seventeen years ago, a new and innovative college of medicine, at Imam Mohammad Ibn Saud University. We had the privilege to create and adopt the most innovative approaches in medical and health professions education. As the college enrolled high school graduates. We thought they have the right to be oriented to these modern instructional strategies. Therefore, we introduced a credited and compulsory learning skills course for the foundation year of all medical students. The course aimed to equip students with essential skills for academic success and lifelong learning in the demanding field of healthcare. However, at the time, the available resources were limited, with most references targeting faculty members rather than medical students. This gap inspired us to dream of creating a dedicated reference book tailored specifically for students. Over time, this dream grew to encompass not just medical students but all students across healthcare professions.

This book, *Essential Learning Skills for Health Professions Students*, is the culmination of years of teaching, research, and collaboration. It brings together insights and expertise from local, regional, and international faculty members representing various healthcare disciplines. Each contributor has been carefully selected for their experience in innovative instructional methods and their commitment to advancing health professions education. Our guiding principle was to ensure that the language, content, and illustrations would remain simple yet engaging, resonating with both undergraduate and graduate students at the foundational level of their programs.

The topics covered in this book reflect the essential skills and challenges that our students have highlighted over the years. From mastering adult learning theories to navigating stress management, critical thinking, and self-directed learning, this book addresses the core needs of healthcare students. The clarity of explanations, practical applications, and visually engaging elements such as illustrations and tables makes this book a practical and user-friendly resource.

We owe a debt of gratitude to our students, whose feedback and experiences shaped the content and approach of this book. To the authors of each chapter, your dedication to sharing your expertise and mentoring the next generation of healthcare professionals has made this project possible. Lastly, we extend our heartfelt thanks to the team at Springer Nature for their exceptional support in bringing this vision to life.

This book represents more than just a guide—it is a legacy of collective experience, a bridge connecting the knowledge of today with the aspirations of tomorrow. We hope it serves as a valuable resource for healthcare students worldwide, empowering them to excel in their studies and contribute meaningfully to building healthier communities.

Riyadh, Saudi Arabia
January 2025

Khalid A. Bin Abdulrahman
Hassan Darami

Introduction

The journey of becoming a healthcare professional is both a privilege and a challenge, marked by rigorous academic demands and the responsibility of preparing for a career dedicated to improving lives. In this rapidly evolving field, mastering essential learning skills is not just a foundation for academic success but a vital tool for lifelong professional development. The healthcare landscape continues to expand in complexity, driven by advances in medical knowledge, technology, and the diverse needs of patient care. For students entering this field, the ability to learn efficiently, adapt to new methodologies, and integrate knowledge into practice is indispensable.

Essential Learning Skills for Health Professions Students has been meticulously designed to address these needs, serving as a comprehensive resource tailored specifically for students in medicine, nursing, and allied health sciences. This textbook fills a critical gap in educational resources, offering guidance that is uniquely aligned with the requirements of health professions education. While many books focus on teaching strategies for instructors or delve into specialized medical content, few resources are dedicated to equipping students with the practical tools needed to thrive in their educational journey and beyond.

A Shifting Paradigm in Health Professions Education

The traditional model of medical and health sciences education, which relied heavily on passive learning and rote memorization, has undergone significant transformation. Today's curricula are characterized by student-centered approaches that emphasize active learning, critical thinking, and the integration of theoretical knowledge with clinical application. Concepts such as problem-based learning, self-directed study, and interdisciplinary teamwork have become central to modern education in the health professions.

Moreover, the shift toward competency-based education places greater responsibility on students to not only acquire knowledge but also demonstrate its practical application. This necessitates mastering a range of learning skills—from effective time management and stress coping mechanisms to advanced communication and presentation abilities. The foundational skills addressed in this textbook are essential not only for academic success but also for the development of professional competence and resilience in the face of the healthcare field's challenges.

Purpose and Goals of This Textbook

This book is designed to serve as both a practical guide and an academic companion for health professions students at various stages of their educational journey. Its primary goal is to empower students with the knowledge and strategies needed to excel in their studies, enhance their clinical performance, and prepare for the lifelong learning required in healthcare careers.

The textbook's structure and content reflect a deep understanding of the unique challenges faced by health professions students. Each chapter is carefully crafted to align with the specific learning outcomes of contemporary medical and health sciences programs. The topics addressed include critical areas such as:

- Active learning and student engagement.
- Problem-based and self-directed learning.
- Time management and productivity.
- Critical and creative thinking.
- Stress management and resilience.
- Effective communication and presentation skills.
- Searching for reliable information and evidence-based practice.

A Unique Approach

What sets this textbook apart is its commitment to practicality and accessibility. The content is presented in a clear and engaging manner, enhanced by illustrative examples, visual aids, and summary boxes that distill key concepts. Real-world applications and case studies provide students with opportunities to connect theoretical principles to their academic and clinical experiences.

Unlike generalized learning resources, *Essential Learning Skills for Health Professions Students* is deeply rooted in the context of healthcare education. It incorporates elements of adult learning theory and active pedagogy, recognizing that health professions students are not just learners but also emerging practitioners who must balance academic responsibilities with clinical training and professional development.

A Global Perspective with Local Relevance

While this textbook addresses the universal principles of learning, it also pays particular attention to the needs and realities of students in the Middle East, specifically Saudi Arabia. Recognizing the cultural and educational nuances of the region, the authors have contextualized key concepts to resonate with local students. For instance, chapters include examples relevant to the healthcare systems and societal expectations of the region, ensuring that the content is not only globally informed but also locally applicable.

This dual focus—global in scope and local in relevance—makes the textbook a valuable resource for diverse audiences. It bridges international best practices with culturally sensitive approaches, offering a unique blend of perspectives that enrich the learning experience.

Preparing for Lifelong Success

Healthcare is an ever-changing field that demands continuous learning and adaptation. The skills and strategies outlined in this book are not limited to the classroom or clinical rotations; they are tools for a lifetime of professional growth. By fostering a mindset of curiosity, resilience, and proactive learning, this textbook prepares students to meet the challenges of their future careers with confidence and competence.

Invitation to the Reader

As you embark on this journey through *Essential Learning Skills for Health Professions Students*, we invite you to approach each chapter with an open mind and a willingness to engage actively with the material. This is more than a textbook; it is a guide to mastering the art and science of learning in one of the most demanding and rewarding professions in the world.

Whether you are an undergraduate starting your first semester or a postgraduate refining your expertise, this book is your companion in developing the skills that will define your success. Welcome to a resource that prioritizes your growth, supports your aspirations, and empowers you to become not only an exceptional student but also an outstanding healthcare professional.

It is our sincere hope that *Essential Learning Skills for Health Professions Students* will serve as a cornerstone in your educational journey, equipping you with the tools and strategies needed to excel in both your academic pursuits and professional endeavors. This textbook is a product of our shared commitment to fostering excellence in health professions education, reflecting a blend of global best practices and regional insights. As educators, we are deeply invested in your growth and success, and we believe that the skills you cultivate here will resonate far beyond your time as a student, shaping you into a confident, compassionate, and competent healthcare professional.

With best regards,

Department of Medical Education,
College of Medicine, Imam Mohammad Ibn
Saud Islamic University (IMSIU)
Riyadh, Saudi Arabia

Khalid A. Bin Abdulrahman

Department of Obstetrics & Gynecology
and Medical Education, College of Medicine
Imam Mohammad Ibn Saud Islamic University (IMSIU)
Riyadh, Saudi Arabia

Hassan Darami

Contents

1 Adult Learning Theories and Their Application in Medical and Health Science Education

Khalid A. Bin Abdulrahman and Somaya Hosny

1.1 Introduction

Health profession education embraces strategies and principles that align with adult learning theories. Understanding and internalizing these principles make it easier for learners to employ strategies and methods that reflect effective learning practices and adapt to the modern techniques and approaches used in teaching and learning across various educational levels in medical and health science schools. Medicine and health sciences are inherently applied professions that require hands-on experience, application, simulation, and practical sessions that support adult learning theories. Although theories might seem abstract and disconnected from medicine, they are integral. This marks the significance of examining the practical applications of theories, which is the primary focus of this chapter.

This chapter delves into the world of adult learning theories and their profound impact on medical and health science education. It explores their historical background, foundational principles, key theoretical models, the challenges and limitations associated with their application in medical education, and emerging perspectives on the future of adult learning. The objectives of this chapter are shown in Box 1.1.

K. A. Bin Abdulrahman (✉)
Department of Medical Education, College of Medicine, Imam Mohammad Ibn Saud Islamic University (IMSIU), Riyadh, Saudi Arabia
e-mail: kab@imamu.edu.sa

S. Hosny
Faculty of Medicine, Suez Canal University, Ismailia, Egypt
e-mail: Somaya@med.suez.edu.eg

K. A. Bin Abdulrahman, H. Darami (eds.), *Essential Learning Skills for Health Professions Students*, https://doi.org/10.1007/978-981-96-5670-7_1

Box 1.1 Objectives of This Chapter

1. Outline the historical background of adult learning theories.
2. Describe the adult learning theories including the main four theories: andragogy, experiential learning, transformative learning, and self-regulated learning.
3. Explain the application of adult learning theories in medicine and health sciences.
4. Discuss the challenges and limitations of using adult learning theories in medical education.
5. List the recommendations for addressing the encountered challenges.

1.2 Historical Background of Adult Learning Theories

The field of adult learning has a rich history, shaped by influential thinkers and evolving perspectives. In the late seventeenth century, John Locke proposed that all our knowledge comes from sensory experiences. In 1911, Edward Thorndike introduced key laws: the "law of effect" (learning from positive outcomes) and the "law of exercise" (repetition strengthens learning). In 1928, Edward Thorndike, along with Bregman, Tilton, and Woodyard, conducted the first systematic investigation of adult learning in their book *Adult Learning* where their foundational work laid the groundwork for understanding how adults learn and how it differs from childhood learning (Thorndike et al. 1928). In the early 1968, Malcolm Knowles introduced the concept of andragogy, a term synonymous with adult education. His work differentiated adult learning from pedagogy (teaching children) and highlighted the importance of individualized approaches for adult learners (Knowles 2015). Over time, other scholars contributed to the understanding of the different adult learning theories which continue to evolve, adapting to technological advancements and cognitive research (Taylor and Hamdy 2013).

1.3 Major Adult Learning Theories and Their Application in Health Sciences

Adult learning theories provide valuable insights into how adults learn and can inform effective teaching practices. By understanding adult learning theory, educators can learn more about the factors that motivate adults to pursue further education. As a result, teachers and trainers can create more meaningful and useful programs for adult learners (Bouchrika 2024).

There is a rich tapestry of theories that illuminate how adults acquire knowledge and skills. These theories include among others the andragogy, self-regulated learning, transformative learning theory, experiential learning theory, project-based learning theory, action learning theory, and collaborative learning theory (Mezirow 1991; Merriam and Bierema 2014).

In this section, four main theories are discussed, namely, andragogy, experiential learning, transformative learning, and self-regulated learning.

1.3.1 Andragogy

Andragogy, one of the most influential learning theories in higher education, was developed by Dr. Malcolm Knowles in 1968. This theory holds particular significance in adult education, especially within the demanding field of medical and health sciences (IGI Global and Information Resources Management Association 2021). Andragogy is founded on four core principles, with self-directed learning being the first. This principle recognizes the autonomy and proactive nature often exhibited by medical professionals, emphasizing their ability to take initiative in managing their own learning process. Advocates of andragogy leverage the principle of self-directed learning to foster engagement through activities like case studies. These activities encourage learners to actively seek solutions, drawing upon their own knowledge and experiences (Halupa 2015). The second principle of andragogy is experience-based learning. Given the practical nature of the medical field, andragogy integrates simulations, clinical rotations, and role-playing scenarios, providing learners with opportunities to apply their knowledge in realistic settings and learn from hands-on experiences. The final principles of andragogy are problem-centered learning and immediate application of knowledge. Considering that real-world medical situations are rarely textbook-perfect, andragogy emphasizes problem-solving skills by presenting learners with elaborate medical cases to analyze and collaboratively work through. Also, in healthcare, timely application of knowledge is crucial. Andragogy ensures the relevance and applicability of acquired knowledge by focusing on learning objectives directly related to real-world scenarios and current medical practices (Halupa 2015). The abovementioned principles of andragogy make it an ideal tool for steering learning in medicine and health sciences. The theory makes its popularity known with the extensive focus on the real-world application of what is learned in classes.

There are multiple techniques that advocates of andragogy propose to be employed in the education of medicine and health sciences. The first technique is the use of case studies. Through case studies, students analyze complex medical cases, using their experience and knowledge to diagnose, propose treatment, and reflect on the learning process (Bridges 2016). The second technique is problem-based learning, in which small groups are tasked with tackling authentic medical scenarios, conducting research, deliberating, and collaborating to find solutions, to foster critical thinking and teamwork. The third technique is the application of clinical rotations in which learners apply theoretical knowledge in actual healthcare settings, thus encountering diverse medical situations directly and refining their practical skills under supervision. The final technique in andragogy is the application of self-directed learning modules. In this technique, tailored modules enable learners to focus on specific areas of interest or address knowledge gaps independently. The modules help to foster self-paced and personalized learning.

Andragogy comes with a range of advantages for learners. The primary advantage is an emphasis on improved knowledge retention. Andragogy emphasizes active participation and application to reinforce understanding (Bridges 2016). Such inputs make information readily accessible during real-world situations. The framework also enables students to improve their critical thinking skills. That is, the framework is based on allowing learners to explore complex scenarios, collaborate on solutions, and reflect on experiences to nurture critical thinking and problem-solving skills. Finally, andragogy is beneficial because it strengthens professional development. Its prospects, such as continuous learning, adaptability to new circumstances, and reflective practice, align with the lifelong learning expected of healthcare professionals.

Figure 1.1 presents the six principles proposed by Malcolm Knowles that can guide educators who wanted to adopt andragogical teaching methods (Wil 2020).

1.3.2 Experiential Learning

Experiential learning is another prevalent framework in medical and health sciences education, recognized for its unique attributes and benefits. Experiential learning theory was developed by David Kolb (Nestel et al. 2023). The theory suggests that learning is a continuous process that involves concrete experiences, reflective observation, abstract conceptualization, and active experimentation (Kolb's four-stage experiential learning cycle is shown in Box 1.2). Educators can include experiential learning in medical and health

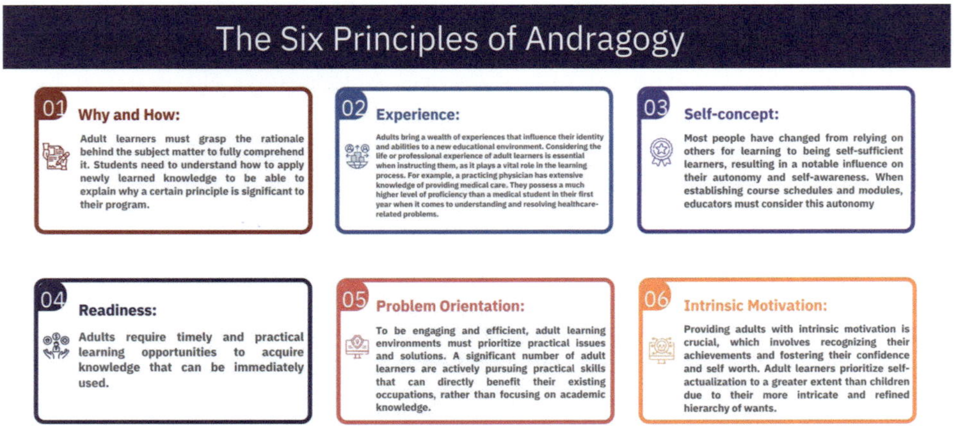

Fig. 1.1 Malcolm Knowles' six principles of andragogy

Box 1.2 Kolb's Four-Stage Experiential Learning Cycle

1. *Concrete Experience*—Students rely mostly on emotions, open-mindedness, and adaptability to handle events and difficulties, rather than using a systematic approach.
2. *Reflective Observation*—Learners form an opinion based on their emotions and thoughts.
3. *Abstract Conceptualization*—Learners rely on methodical planning and constructive concepts and theories to address practical concerns and problems.
4. *Active Experimentation*—Learners engage in active learning by conducting experiments in various circumstances, adopting a practical approach rather than passively observing.

science education through clinical rotations, internships, simulations, and hands-on laboratory activities. These experiences help students apply their theoretical knowledge to real-world circumstances while reflecting on their practice.

The application of experiential learning is based on specific principles. The first principle is learning by doing. This principle focuses on the understanding that medical professionals require hands-on skills and rapid decision-making abilities (Swanwick 2019). Experiential learning facilitates this by immersing learners in simulated or real-world settings, such as high-fidelity simulations where learners engage in clinical procedures and decision-making within realistic scenarios using mannequins and actors. It also encourages standardized patient encounters where actors can portray specific medical conditions, enabling learners to refine their communication skills, history, and physical examination. Learning by doing also encourages clinical rotations in which learners can interact with patients under supervision. Such interactions will give them invaluable hands-on experience and exposure to various medical cases.

The second principle of experiential learning is reflection on experience. Proponents of this approach argue that mere participation in activities is insufficient for deep learning. To address this, the framework incorporates debriefing and reflective practices following each experience, allowing learners to derive meaningful insights and enhance their understanding (Nestel et al. 2023). Activities within this principle include group discussions where students can analyze the successes, challenges, and decision-making processes. The principle also focuses on individual journaling to prompt self-reflection on gained learning and areas for improvement. Finally, learners can participate in video reviews of simulation performances for targeted feedback and self-assessment.

The final principle of experiential learning is to emphasize illustrations within learning settings. In simulation labs, students practice complex procedures, such as cardiopulmonary resuscitation, intubation, or surgical techniques in controlled environments, receiving immediate feedback to refine their skills (Swanwick 2019). The principle also fosters role-playing scenarios that cover communication challenges, ethical dilemmas, or delivering difficult news to equip learners with empathy, communication skills, and the ability to navigate challenging situations. The theory also allows students to participate in community health initiatives to provide real-world experience, foster social responsibility, and demonstrate the impacts of their future profession. Finally, there are facilitated discussions following simulations or clinical encounters to encourage critical thinking, analysis, and a deeper understanding of the learning experience.

Experiential learning offers a variety of advantages, making it highly effective in educational settings. One key benefit is its ability to enhance the development of practical skills among learners. By engaging in hands-on practice within realistic settings, students can refine their technical abilities, build confidence, and prepare for real-world clinical scenarios (Nestel et al. 2023). Additionally, experiential learning fosters critical thinking skills by encouraging students to reflect on their decisions and evaluate outcomes. This reflective process promotes problem-solving abilities and critical reasoning, which are vital for effective medical practice. Finally, experiential learning promotes teamwork and communication. Collaborative learning experiences in simulations or clinical settings cultivate teamwork, communication skills, and the ability to learn from peers (Swanwick 2019). The abovementioned benefits have marked the popularity of experiential learning initiatives in contemporary learning settings of the medical and health sciences.

1.3.3 Self-Regulated Learning (SRL)

SRL is another vital framework for enhancing learning and knowledge acquisition in present-day medicine and health sciences learning institutions. This theory focuses on controlling learners' cognition, motivation, and behavior to achieve their learning objectives (Bastable 2017). Medical and health science educators can help students learn independently by offering scaffolding, feedback, and metacognitive methods. Also, students can learn to establish precise learning objectives, track their progress, request assistance when necessary, and reflect on their learning practices.

The application of self-regulated learning emphasizes several key principles, the first being metacognition. This principle encourages learners to develop an awareness of their learning processes, enabling them to identify their strengths and address their weaknesses effectively (Mu and Hatch 2022). In this principle, learners can discern when they grasp a concept or when further clarification is necessary and decide which strategies are most effective. The second principle is the setting and planning goals, in which learners are encouraged to establish precise, attainable learning objectives and adapt their study plans accordingly (Bastable 2017). The strategy involves breaking down complex tasks, effectively prioritizing, and allocating adequate time for learning activities.

The third principle of SRL is monitoring and evaluation. This principle involves learners actively assessing their progress, evaluating their understanding, and identifying areas for improvement. Strategies may include regular self-assessments, seeking feedback from mentors, and reflecting on performance during practical exercises (Dickman and Schuster 2020).

Finally, SRL focuses on self-motivation and regulation. The model allows learners to maintain internal motivation and employ tactics to overcome obstacles and distractions. This might involve time management strategies, cultivating a conducive learning environment, and rewarding progress.

SRL has been applied in various aspects of education within medicine and health sciences institutions. First, among the applications are personalized learning plans. In the plans, students devise customized study plans based on their learning preferences, strengths, and areas that need improvement, fostering self-awareness and focused learning endeavors (Dickman and Schuster 2020). SRL also constitutes reflective journaling to encourage learners to consider their learning journeys, identify achievements and obstacles, and set feasible future goals. In addition, SRL stimulates the application of peer learning groups (Mu and Hatch 2022). SRL proponents believe that collaborative learning environments enable students to explore complex topics, elucidate concepts with one another, and receive constructive feedback, promoting self-assessment and knowledge integration. Finally, SRL comes with technology-assisted learning. Educational applications, adaptive learning platforms, and online resources empower learners to customize their learning pace, monitor progress, and access targeted materials, nurturing self-directed learning.

In general, proficiency in SRL equips learners with the means to continually adapt, update their knowledge, and stay current in the ever-changing world of medicine throughout their careers. Additionally, it increases knowledge retention (Dickman and Schuster 2020). Active monitoring, reflection, and personalized learning methodologies result in deeper comprehension and superior knowledge retention compared to passive learning approaches. Finally, this learning technique is characterized by enhanced decision-making and problem-solving. Effective self-regulation cultivates critical thinking and the ability to autonomously analyze situations, design solutions, and make informed decisions in dynamic clinical environments. The following figure (Fig. 1.2) shows the self-regulated learning cycle.

1.3.4 Transformative Learning

Transformative learning is a learner-centered approach that actively engages students through critical reflection and meaningful discourse. It encourages learners to challenge assumptions and reexamine expectations, fostering deeper understanding and shifts in perspective that inform and guide future actions (Kleinheksel 2014). Transformative learning stimulates the development of competence and self-confidence in new roles and relationships that bring about change in the learning and working environments (Tsimane and Downing 2020).

Transformative learning theory, developed by American sociologist Jack Mezirow in the late 1970s, explains how adults undergo profound shifts in their understanding of the world. It centers around shifting our mental "frame of reference"—the lens through which

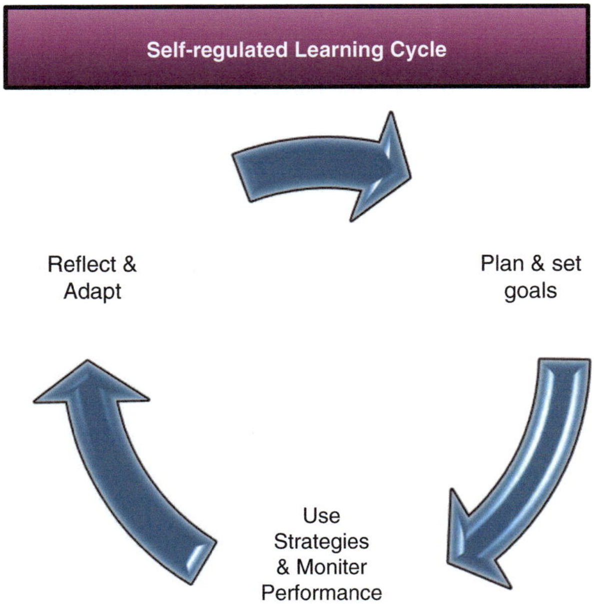

Fig. 1.2 Self-regulated learning cycle

we perceive reality. It involves profound changes in our understanding, beliefs, and perspectives, leading to personal growth and expanded awareness (Mezirow 1991). Mezirow believed that adults do not merely apply old knowledge to new experiences; instead, they engage in critical evaluation and self-assessment, leading to a reframing of their beliefs and values.

As described by Mezirow, the frame of reference is a mental filter that influences how we experience the world. It is composed of two parts, the first is *habits of mind*, which is deeply ingrained patterns of thinking, feeling, and acting. These are tough to change. Example of a habit of mind is ethnocentrism (the belief in one's ethnicity's superiority). The second part is the *points of view*, which is derived from broader habits of mind. An example of a perspective is the Western tradition of serving beverages with ice, which reflects a broader cultural inclination rooted in national identity. Contrary to habits of mind, points of view are more malleable; its focus lies in altering our mental perspective—the lens through which we view reality (Mezirow 1991).

There are ten phases for transformative learning as identified in Mezirow's 1978 original study. The phases are as follows:

1. *Disorienting dilemma*: an event or experience that disrupts existing beliefs and assumptions
2. *Self-examination*: reflecting on our assumptions and values
3. *Critical assessment*: evaluating our habitual ways of thinking
4. *Recognition of a connection*: identifying shared experiences or perspectives with others
5. *Exploration of options*: considering alternative viewpoints and potential new directions

6. *Planning for action*: developing a strategy to implement meaningful change
7. *Acquisition of knowledge*: gaining new information or skills to support transformation
8. *Trying of new roles*: experimenting with new behaviors in a safe context
9. *Building competence and self-confidence*: gaining confidence in our transformed self
10. *Reintegration into life*: applying the new perspective in daily life (Mezirow 1991).

The following figure (Fig. 1.3) shows the ten phases of transformational learning theory, as described by Mezirow.

There are different points of view regarding transformative learning other than that suggested by Mezirow (1991). Although Mezirow believed that discourse with others is important in transformative learning, Cranton (2006) reported that it can occur without discourse. Mezirow (1991) considered the transformative learning as rational and objective. However, Dirkx and Mezirow (2006) suggested that emotions and the unconscious have influence on transformation learning. While Mezirow identified ten phases for transformative learning, Tennant and Pogson (1995) suggested that changes in beliefs might simply be part of the natural life cycles of development. Newman (2012) pondered whether true transformation even exists, suggesting that these changes might merely be the outcome of effective learning. Transformative learning theory has important implications for educational practice, particularly in higher education. This includes curriculum design, teaching strategies, assessment, and professional development.

Through implementing transformative learning, educators can design curricula that encourage students to critically reflect on their assumptions and beliefs (Mezirow 1991). Additionally, introducing scenarios that challenge students' existing perspectives can

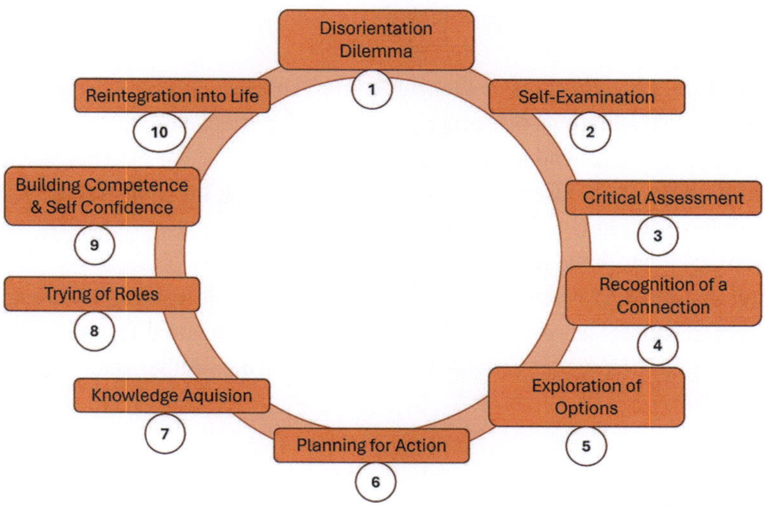

Fig. 1.3 Mezirow's ten phases of transformational learning

stimulate transformative learning. For example, case studies that present ethical dilemmas can encourage students to reassess their professional values and beliefs (Cranton 2006).

Creating a classroom environment that encourages open dialogue and critical discourse is vital for transformative learning. Educators should employ diverse strategies to foster a culture of inquiry and reflection, such as facilitating group discussions, organizing debates, and encouraging collaborative problem-solving activities. These approaches create opportunities for students to question assumptions, share perspectives, and engage in meaningful reflection (Brookfield 2012).

Providing support helps learners navigate the often challenging process of transformation. Thus, educators should take time to know students as individuals, recognizing their preferences and engaging them in a variety of approaches that foster transformative learning. This can be done through one-to-one mentoring, feedback sessions, and support groups (Taylor 2008).

Furthermore, assessments that require students to reflect on their learning experiences and articulate changes in their perspectives such as reflective essays, portfolios, and self-assessment reports can be used as powerful tools (King 2009). Conducting continuous, formative assessment helps learners understand their progress and areas for improvement. Mackintosh-Franklin reported that regular formative assessment facilitates and transform learning (Mackintosh-Franklin 2021).

Scholars have extensively explored transformative learning over the past 45 years where transformative learning has evolved into a mature collection of theories. Their research has illuminated transformative learning relevance in contemporary contexts, revealing how it intersects with diverse fields and enhances human adaptability and growth (Hoggan and Finnegan 2023).

After exploring various adult learning theories, it becomes evident that they underscore several fundamental principles. These include the following (Palis and Quiros 2014):

- Clear goals and objectives for any teaching intervention.
- Relevance to real situations of learner's everyday experience.
- Building on experience and learner's prior knowledge.
- Reflection on the learning process by learners, including how they learn, what strategies work best, and how to improve themselves.
- Active engagement in the learning process.
- Teaching that prioritizes learners taking into account adult learning theories, enabling instructors to address learners' needs, objectives, and contextual factors.
- Teacher is a facilitator that provide guidance to learners rather than merely transfer knowledge.

1.4 Challenges and Limitations of Incorporating Adult Learning Theories in Medical Education

Incorporating adult learning theories into medical education presents various challenges and limitations. The reported challenges include the following:

- *Time constraints*: Medical curricula are often packed with content, leaving limited time for in-depth exploration of adult learning principles; this time constraints conflict with the thoroughness of educational methods (IGI Global and Information Resources Management Association 2021).
- *Limited resources*: This hinders the use of adequate teaching and learning facilities (Bridges 2016).
- *Diverse learner backgrounds*: Medical students come from diverse backgrounds, with varying prior knowledge and experiences. Tailoring instruction to meet these individual needs can be challenging (Merriam et al. 2007).
- *Clinical demands*: Medical education occurs within the context of clinical practice. Balancing clinical responsibilities with learning activities poses a constraint (Merriam et al. 2007).
- *Assessment challenges*: Designing assessments that align with adult learning principles can be complex. Traditional exams may not capture deeper understanding or reflective thinking (Taylor and Hamdy 2013).
- *Faculty development*: Faculty development must help educators in promoting effective teaching practices and lifelong learning among students. Lack of faculty development hinders successful implementation of adult learning theories (Taylor and Hamdy 2013). Faculty development must help educators in promoting

To address the previous reported challenges, medical schools should invest in faculty development programs that emphasize adult learning theories and their practical application, encourage ongoing professional development for educators, integrate adult learning principles into curricular planning and design, and foster collaboration between educators, clinicians, and curriculum committees. Additionally, medical schools should use multiple assessment methods that align with adult learning processes.

1.5 Summary

Adapting to the evolving landscape of medicine and health sciences is crucial for educational institutions. In this context, theories such as andragogy, experiential learning, self-regulated learning, and transformative learning provide valuable frameworks to address current educational demands. Each of these theories offers distinct principles that make them highly relevant to modern education, promoting deeper learning, critical thinking, and self-directed growth. However, their implementation is not without challenges.

Institutions often face constraints such as limited resources, time pressures, clinical demands, assessment difficulties, and a lack of professional development opportunities for educators. These barriers must be addressed to fully utilize the potential of these learning theories in shaping the future of medical and health sciences education. Incorporating adult learning theories into medical education requires a delicate balance. By recognizing the challenges and proactively addressing them, educators can foster a more effective, learner-centered environment that promotes deeper engagement and meaningful learning.

References

Bastable SB. Essentials of patient education. 2nd ed. Burlington: John & Bartlett Learning; 2017.

Bouchrika I. Adult learning theory in 2024: methods and techniques of teaching adults. Education. 2024.

Bridges S. Educational technologies in medical and health sciences education. Cham: Springer; 2016.

Brookfield SD. Teaching for critical thinking: tools and techniques to help students question their assumptions. San Francisco: Jossey-Bass; 2012.

Cranton P. Understanding and promoting transformative learning: a guide for educators of adults. 2nd ed. San Francisco: Jossey-Bass; 2006.

Dickman N, Schuster B. Active education for future doctors. Cham: Springer; 2020.

Dirkx JM, Mezirow J. Musings and reflections on the meaning, context, and process of transformative learning: a dialogue between John M. Dirkx and Jack Mezirow. J Transform Educ. 2006;4:123–39.

Halupa C. (Ed.). Transformative curriculum design in health sciences education. Medical Information Science Reference an imprint of IGI Global; 2015 https://doi.org/10.4018/978-1-4666-8571-0.

Hoggan C, Finnegan F. Transformative learning theory: where we are after 45 years. New Dir Adult Contin Educ. 2023;177:5–11. https://doi.org/10.1002/ace.20474.

IGI Global, Information Resources Management Association. Research anthology on adult education and the development of lifelong learners. Hershey: IGI Global; 2021.

King KP. Handbook of the evolving research of transformative learning based on the learning activities survey. Charlotte: Information Age Publishing; 2009.

Kleinheksel AJ. Transformative learning through virtual patient simulations: predicting critical student reflections. Clin Simul Nurs. 2014;10(6):e301–8.

Knowles MS. The adult learner: the definitive classic in adult education and human resource development. Oxon: Routledge; 2015.

Mackintosh-Franklin C. An evaluation of formative feedback and its impact on undergraduate student nurse academic achievement. Nurse Educ Pract. 2021;50:102930. https://doi.org/10.1016/j.nepr.2020.102930.

Merriam SB, Bierema LL. Adult learning: linking theory and practice. Wiley; 2014.

Merriam SB, Caffarella RS, Baumgartner LM. Learning in adulthood: a comprehensive guide. 3rd ed. John Wiley & Sons; 2007.

Mezirow J. Transformative dimensions of adult learning. San Francisco: Jossey-Bass; 1991.

Mu F, Hatch J. Adult learning and decision making an integrated theory. Singapore: World Scientific; 2022.

Nestel D, Reedy G, McKenna L, Gough S. Clinical education for the health professions: theory and practice. Singapore: Springer; 2023.

Newman F. The myth of transformative learning. Change. 2012;44(6):24–9.

Palis AG, Quiros PA. Adult learning principles and presentation pearls. Middle East Afr J Ophthalmol. 2014;21(2):114–22.

Swanwick T. Understanding medical education: evidence theory and practice. 3rd ed. Hoboken: Wiley Blackwell; 2019.

Taylor EW. Transformative learning theory. New Dir Adult Contin Educ. 2008;(119):5–15.

Taylor DCM, Hamdy H. Adult learning theories: implications for learning and teaching in medical education: AMEE Guide No. 83. Med Teach. 2013;35(11):e1561–72. https://doi.org/10.3109/0142159X.2013.828153.

Tennant M, Pogson P. Learning and change in the adult years: a developmental perspective. San Francisco: Jossey-Bass; 1995.

Thorndike EL, Bregman EO, Tilton JW, & Woodyard E. (1928). Adult learning. The Macmillan Company, New York, NY.

Tsimane TA, Downing C. Transformative learning in nursing education: a concept analysis. Int J Nurs Sci. 2020;7:91–8.

Wil. Six principles of andragogy. Malcolm Knowles; 2020.

2 Attitudes and Practices of a Professional Health Science Student

Khalid A. Bin Abdulrahman, Abdulaziz Fahd Alkaabba, Osama A. Alkhamees, and Salah-Ud-Din Khan

Learning Objectives

1. *Define and describe medical professionalism.*
   Learners will be able to define medical professionalism and identify its core elements, including politeness, humility, truthfulness, competence, and respect for patient autonomy.
2. *Apply ethical principles in healthcare settings.*
   Learners will demonstrate the ability to integrate ethical considerations, including Islamic ethics and advocacy for health equity, in addressing complex dilemmas and promoting patient rights and dignity.
3. *Develop professional identity and essential behaviours.*
   Learners will evaluate and enhance their professional identity by adopting key behaviours such as punctuality, integrity, effective communication, and lifelong learning, fostering positive interactions in both academic and clinical environments.

K. A. Bin Abdulrahman (✉)
Department of Medical Education, College of Medicine, Imam Mohammad Ibn Saud Islamic University (IMSIU), Riyadh, Saudi Arabia
e-mail: kab@imamu.edu.sa

A. F. Alkaabba
Department of Family and Community Medicine, College of Medicine, Imam Mohammad Ibn Saud Islamic University (IMSIU), Riyadh, Saudi Arabia
e-mail: afkaabba@imamu.edu.sa

O. A. Alkhamees
Department of Pharmacology, College of Medicine, Imam Mohammad Ibn Saud Islamic University (IMSIU), Riyadh, Saudi Arabia
e-mail: oakhamees@imamu.edu.sa

S. Khan
Department of Biochemistry, College of Medicine, Imam Mohammad Ibn Saud Islamic University (IMSIU), Riyadh, Saudi Arabia
e-mail: sdikhan@imamu.edu.sa

K. A. Bin Abdulrahman, H. Darami (eds.), *Essential Learning Skills for Health Professions Students*, https://doi.org/10.1007/978-981-96-5670-7_2

2.1 Introduction

Physician professionalism is a vital concept that plays a crucial role in the healthcare system, as it directly influences patients' well-being and protects their rights. The attitudes, feelings, and behaviours of health science students are instrumental in shaping their future conduct as lawful, ethical, accountable, and equitable healthcare professionals. This chapter presents an overview of medical professionalism and its core elements, which include politeness towards patients, humility, truthfulness, and competence. Additionally, it addresses negative behaviours that can undermine these principles, such as cheating, inappropriate attire, rudeness, and plagiarism. Understanding these detrimental practices and their consequences is essential for students to avoid them and strive for excellence in their careers.

Conversely, this chapter emphasizes the essential behaviours that healthcare students should adopt, including punctuality, integrity, respect for patient autonomy, and effective communication skills. Upholding these standards equips students with a solid foundation for successful and rewarding careers in the healthcare field. This chapter delineates the attitudes and behaviours expected of professional health science students and illustrates their roles within the healthcare delivery system through a comprehensive analysis of the aforementioned topics.

2.2 Medical Professionalism

Medical professionalism includes the values, beliefs, and standards essential for maintaining the integrity of the medical field and delivering quality healthcare. Acknowledging the primacy of the social contract—known as the trust model (TM)—is crucial for the medical profession to evolve and maintain public trust. Thus, medical professionalism involves honouring ethical principles and acting responsibly, morally, and ethically towards patients and fellow professionals. This respect is reflected in honouring patients' rights, autonomy, independence, privacy, and cultural preferences. Kindness in healthcare includes courtesy, empathy, and responsiveness to patients' concerns and needs.

Integrity is another cornerstone of medical professionalism, ensuring that healthcare providers adhere to ethical standards and practice honesty in all professional dealings. This entails not misleading patients, clearly explaining their conditions, and being transparent about treatment options. Integrity also extends to interactions with colleagues, supervisors, and other stakeholders in the healthcare system, as well as promoting truthfulness and adherence to corporate ethics.

Competency is equally vital, and ongoing education and professional development are necessary for providing high-quality healthcare. Healthcare professionals must stay informed about advancements in science and technology, engaging in formal training as well as practical experiences such as workshops and seminars.

Collaboration is another key aspect of professionalism in healthcare. Stakeholders must promote interprofessional teamwork to develop effective care delivery plans. Such cooperation not only increases the quality of patient care but also fosters a positive work environment characterized by mutual respect and dignity. Effective communication and courtesy are crucial for achieving team goals and building trust with patients, as a respectful environment encourages patient compliance with medical advice and treatment regimens.

Moreover, medical professionalism is closely tied to ethical considerations. Ethical management is vital for healthcare facilities and practitioners, who often face complex ethical dilemmas that require sound guidance. Adhering to ethical principles helps ensure that patient rights and dignity are respected, thereby reducing corruption and upholding the integrity of the healthcare profession.

In addition to professional expertise, medical professionalism involves a commitment to altruism and advocacy. Healthcare providers are expected to prioritize their patients' welfare over their own, reflecting the dedication inherent in their roles. Advocacy involves healthcare professionals championing both individual and collective patient needs, as well as broader social justice issues that impact patient care. This form of professionalism positions providers as change agents and leaders in promoting health equity.

2.3 Essential Components of Medical Professionalism

Medical professionalism is a cornerstone of ethical and exemplary patient care and is built upon a foundation of core principles. At its heart lies a profound respect for patient autonomy, dignity, and cultural diversity, and self-determination is recognized as an inviolable value. By placing patients at the centre of care and honouring their choices, healthcare providers foster trust, increase satisfaction, and empower individuals to actively participate in their healthcare journey. This patient-centred approach is pivotal in cultivating a collaborative partnership between patients and providers, leading to improved health outcomes (Beauchamp and Childress 2019).

Compassion, a fundamental attribute of effective healthcare, is essential for alleviating patient suffering and building trust. It includes both physical and emotional care, recognizing the holistic nature of patient well-being. When patients feel understood and valued, they are more likely to engage in their treatment plan and experience positive health outcomes.

Integrity is the bedrock of trust in the healthcare profession. By adhering to ethical standards and maintaining honesty, healthcare providers foster a culture of reliability and accountability (Cruess and Cruess 2014). This trust is essential for effective collaboration among healthcare teams and for building strong patient–provider relationships.

Lifelong learning is indispensable for maintaining competence in a rapidly evolving healthcare landscape. By staying abreast of scientific advancements and clinical best practices, healthcare professionals ensure that they deliver optimal care to their patients.

Continuing education, certifications, and specialized training contribute to the delivery of high-quality care and improve problem-solving abilities in complex clinical situations (Epstein 2002).

Effective teamwork is essential for delivering patient-centred care. Despite shared standards of practice in the medical field, many medical professionals lack formal training in effective teaching skills. Thus, the professional development of medical educators is essential, as it involves unique knowledge and skills parallel to those of medical practice. By fostering open communication and collaboration among healthcare providers, as well as involving patients and their families, healthcare teams can develop comprehensive treatment plans that address the whole person (Glicken and Merenstein 2007). This collaborative approach increases patient satisfaction, improves outcomes, and creates a supportive environment for patients and their caregivers.

In summary, medical professionalism is a dynamic and multifaceted construct that requires ongoing commitment and reflection. By embodying these core principles—respect, compassion, integrity, competence, and teamwork—healthcare professionals can deliver exceptional care, build strong patient relationships, and contribute to the overall health and well-being of their communities. Furthermore, professionalism transcends technical and clinical competencies by including advocacy and social responsibility. Healthcare professionals are uniquely positioned to act as leaders and advocates for community well-being. This role involves addressing issues related to patient care, such as access to services, education, and socioeconomic challenges. Through advocacy, healthcare providers can drive significant changes in the healthcare delivery system, promoting equitable access for marginalized populations. Figure 2.1 summarizes the essential components of medical professionalism.

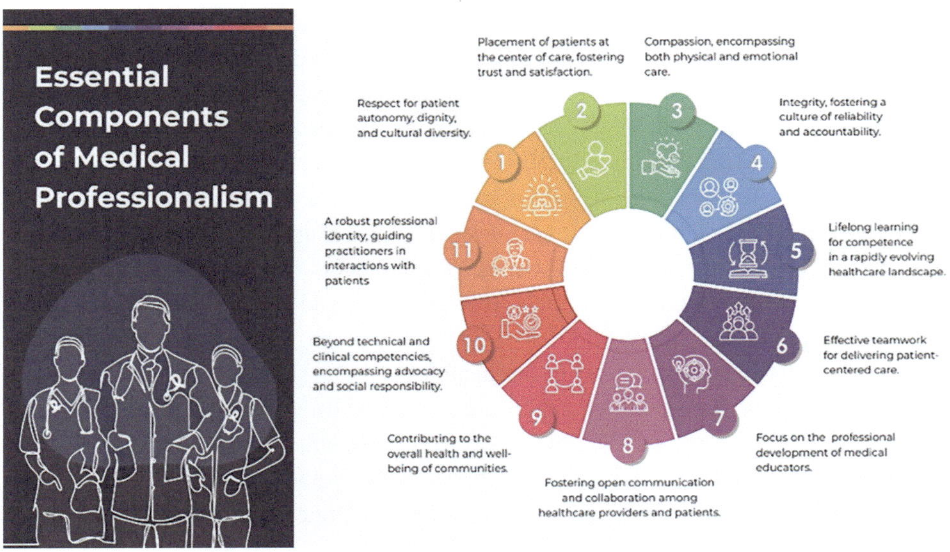

Fig. 2.1 Essential components of medical professionalism

A robust professional identity is the cornerstone upon which healthcare students can build successful and fulfilling careers. It involves a complex interplay of values, beliefs, and behaviours that guide practitioners in their interactions with patients, colleagues, and the broader healthcare system. This chapter examines the essential components of professional identity, explores their significance in the context of healthcare, and provides practical strategies for their cultivation.

2.4 Core Components of Professional Identity

A robust professional identity in healthcare is grounded in several fundamental principles (Hussein and Kaabba 2015; American Board of Medical Specialties Board of Directors 2012). At its core lies *respect* for the inherent dignity and autonomy of every individual, irrespective of background or circumstances. This principle, which is deeply rooted in Islamic teachings emphasizing the sanctity of life and compassionate treatment, is the cornerstone of patient-centred care. Healthcare professionals must also uphold the highest standards of *integrity*, characterized by honesty, trustworthiness, and adherence to ethical principles. Aligned with Islamic values of truthfulness and reliability, integrity fosters trust and ensures ethical conduct.

To deliver optimal patient care, *competence* is essential. This involves a lifelong commitment to acquiring and applying knowledge and skills. The Islamic emphasis on seeking knowledge and striving for excellence underscores the importance of continuous learning and professional development. Effective *teamwork* is equally crucial, as it facilitates collaboration among healthcare professionals from diverse backgrounds. Islamic principles of cooperation and mutual support create a harmonious environment conducive to shared decision-making and patient-centred care.

A profound sense of *altruism* is intrinsic to the healthcare profession. Prioritizing the well-being of patients and contributing to the betterment of society align with the Islamic value of service to humanity. Healthcare professionals with a strong altruistic inclination are motivated to go beyond their clinical duties to advocate for the health and well-being of their patients and communities. This leads to *advocacy* for patient rights, health equity, and positive healthcare policy changes, a responsibility that resonates with the Islamic imperative to uphold justice and support vulnerable populations.

By embodying these core principles, healthcare professionals cultivate a strong professional identity that is both ethically sound and spiritually grounded. This identity empowers them to deliver exceptional patient care, build trust, and contribute meaningfully to the health and well-being of their communities.

2.5 Islamic Ethics: A Moral Compass

The practice of medicine is inherently intertwined with ethical considerations. Ethical frameworks, including Islamic ethics and other moral philosophies, provide guidance for navigating complex healthcare dilemmas. For example, principles such as beneficence (doing good), nonmaleficence (avoiding harm), and justice (ensuring fairness) are universal concepts that underpin ethical decision-making in healthcare.

In Islam, seeking medical care is vital for preserving life and requires medical knowledge. Imam Shafi'i (d. 204H/820 CE) stressed knowledge in two areas: religion and the human body. Muslims share a responsibility to cultivate the practice of healthcare. Al Izz ibn Abdul Salam (d. 660H/1243 CE) likened medicine's purpose to that of Islamic law ('Shari'ah') in his book *Qawa'id al Ahkam*, as both aim at obtaining human benefit through health and safety. He adds that medicine aims to maintain health, restore health, or minimize health issues, even if it means accepting a lesser harm (Ali and Chamsi-Pasha 2015).

The *Quran* and Prophet Muhammad's (PBUH) teachings guide doctor–patient ethics. The Prophet offered guidance on seeking medical help and patient consent. Islamic jurists require qualified, licenced practitioners who obtain patient consent (or guardian consent if needed). The *Quran* and Sunnah emphasize good 'khuluq' (manners) for Muslim doctors, including mercy, patience, and honesty (Arawi 2011).

The bedrock of ethical healthcare practice lies in the integration of ethical principles. Integrating these principles not only elevates the quality of care but also strengthens the moral compass of the healthcare community. To navigate the intricate ethical dilemmas that inevitably arise in healthcare, students must familiarize themselves with these fundamental guidelines.

The infusion of Islamic ethics into the professional identity of healthcare practitioners provides a robust framework for guiding clinical decisions (Hedayat and Pirzadeh 2001; Padela 2007). Central to this ethical framework is the unwavering respect for the inherent dignity and worth of every human life. This principle underpins the imperative to deliver just and equitable care to all patients, irrespective of their socioeconomic status or background. Healthcare professionals must actively strive to promote the well-being of their patients while diligently working to prevent harm. The principle of nonmaleficence dictates the avoidance of harm and the minimization of potential risks associated with treatment. Finally, the cornerstone of patient-centred care is respect for patient autonomy, which empowers individuals to make informed decisions about their healthcare journey. By embracing these ethical principles, healthcare professionals can cultivate practices rooted in compassion, integrity, and the pursuit of optimal patient outcomes. These ethical principles align seamlessly with the core components of professional identity and provide a robust framework for healthcare practice. By integrating Islamic ethics into their professional lives, healthcare practitioners can make informed and compassionate decisions (Athar et al. 2005; Kasule 2010).

It is also essential to emphasize that these principles are meant to be applied within the remits and limits of the society in which the healthcare provider works. In other words, these principles must be respected but must also be adjusted appropriately for the local context, which will differ from one place to another.

2.6 Cultivating a Strong Professional Identity

The development of a robust professional identity in healthcare is an ongoing journey that necessitates deliberate self-reflection and action. Healthcare students can foster this identity by cultivating a strong professional demeanour that includes appropriate attire, timely behaviour, and respectful communication. This approach establishes a foundation of trust and contributes to a positive healthcare environment. A robust ethical compass, grounded in Islamic principles and aligned with professional standards, is essential for navigating the complex moral dilemmas inherent in healthcare. Engaging in discussions and case studies can enhance ethical decision-making capabilities.

Lifelong learning is paramount in the dynamic healthcare landscape. Healthcare professionals must continually seek knowledge and engage in professional development to maintain competence and deliver optimal patient care. Placing the patient at the core of care is fundamental. Building strong therapeutic relationships through active listening and empathy fosters patient satisfaction and adherence to treatment plans. Effective collaboration among healthcare professionals is essential for delivering high-quality care and is highly appreciated by medical students (Adkoli et al. 2011; AlKhater 2021). Fostering teamwork, open communication, and mutual respect improves care coordination and strengthens one's overall professional identity. Seeking mentorship from experienced healthcare professionals provides invaluable guidance, support, and insights into professional growth. Engaging in community service demonstrates a commitment to altruism and compassion, further enriching one's professional identity. Figure 2.2 demonstrates the professional identity of healthcare.

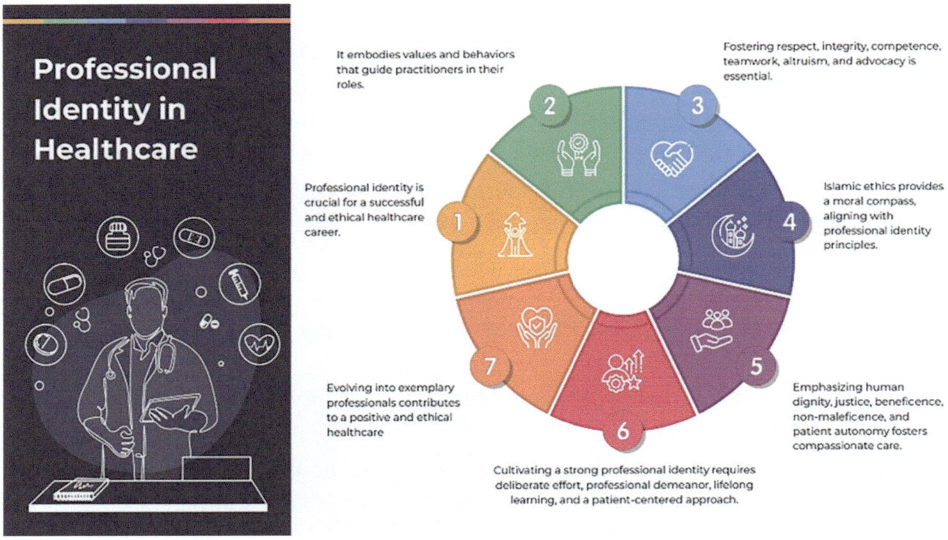

Fig. 2.2 Professional identity of healthcare

2.7 Unwanted Attitudes and Practices Among Medical Students

It is rather disheartening that some of the behaviours and conduct of the medical students here are below par with those of the profession and hinder the improvement of health and care services in the country. First, one must acknowledge that cheating is an immediate threat to these priorities. Cheating also affects the learning system, which supports the knowledge and quality work required in patient care (Epstein and Hundert 2002). Cheating erodes the quality of education and threatens patient safety due to the admission of unqualified professionals in the health field.

Some supporting information should be highlighted. First, when students cheat, they harm themselves because they do not assimilate the knowledge and skills necessary to improve patients' lives, which has detrimental effects when the cheaters become practising doctors. They may not have adequate skills and knowledge for providing healthcare services, which exposes clients to the risk of being misdiagnosed or offered the wrong treatment. Furthermore, cheating creates a dishonest environment that will follow students in their further professional activities concerning teamwork, trust, and, consequently, the quality of patient treatment.

Failure to follow the dress code can be associated with negligence and carelessness in anything one does. Patients' dressing and state of hygiene also affect their perception of the quality of health service delivery and may even lead them to question the professionalism of health facilities or personnel. Work uniforms indicate how seriously a professional takes the job, and those in the healthcare sector regard uniforms as significant, as they indicate one's respect for the noble profession one is practising. Professional dress lays the groundwork for patient relations and plays a major role in determining patients' level of confidence and trust in any caregiver. Punctuality complements the aspects of professional dress, as well as establishing proper tone and indicating professional handling of patients. The social importance of punctuality is evident regarding time management between patients and doctors because timely actions and treatments improve patients' conditions.

An additional example of poor academic conduct is plagiarism, which directly defeats the idea of a person's academic development and violates all the principles of academic integrity. There are several constructive practices whereby health science students are expected to develop new ideas, namely, inclusion and referencing, to ensure that the work of other individuals has been acknowledged (Glicken and Merenstein 2007). The misuse of others' work is not only academically unproductive but also an example of ethical wrongdoing that follows an individual in their practice; therefore, there are severe consequences. Additionally, plagiarism is a form of cheating. It often leads to the subversion of the values of hard intellectual work and to the erosion of trust between professionals and their peers, clinicians, and clients.

Additionally, undesirable behaviours such as impoliteness, lack of courtesy, and other aspects of interpersonal communication can be detrimental to providing effective and safe patient care. Discourteous or noncourteous communication in interactions with patients can decrease patients' compliance with the care plans established by the doctors. Empathy is lacking, and patients may feel that their care providers do not understand or care about them, which can result in poor health outcomes and dissatisfaction with the healthcare system.

2.8 Consequences of Unwanted Practices

The outcomes of unwanted practices adopted by medical students are dire. First, rudeness and impropriety significantly reduce clients' confidence in the healthcare team; hence, the patient–provider relationship is damaged. Engagement is critical to the healthcare delivery system because trust is a critical component, and loss of trust may lead to low patient compliance and dissatisfaction. Second, effective practices improve the quality of care given to patients in hospitals and other health units. A good example of how these negative behaviours can have a knock-on effect on patient care is that when healthcare workers are involved in scandals such as cheating or poor punctuality, the standard of care delivery to patients is affected in equal measure; this may bring about harm in one way or another and result in poorer levels of health among the targeted patients.

Moreover, unprofessionalism can cause much harm to both the person and the reputable institution at which the person is employed. This type of damage cannot be overemphasized. It affects the future employment of the person involved and the credibility of the institution. Credibility depends on cultivating patient trust; therefore, professionalism is crucial, as the quality of care services affects an institution's reputable professional image. Figure 2.3 summarizes the unwanted attitudes and practices among medical students.

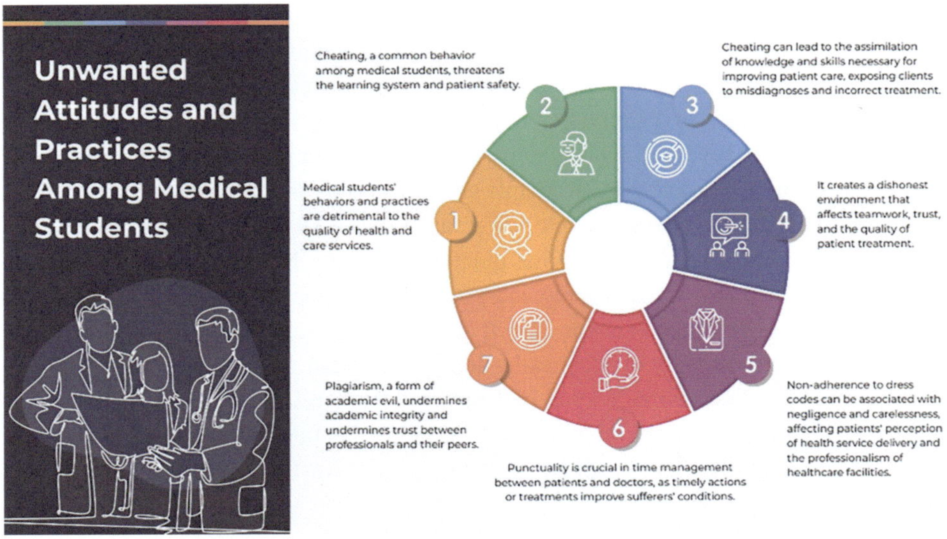

Fig. 2.3 Unwanted attitudes and practices among medical students

2.9 Typical Professional Behaviour of Healthcare Students

The role of health practitioners in society and the community is unique and essential, which is why it is crucial for students in the field to maintain professionalism. As future health professionals, students acquire distinctive skills that not only empower them to provide high-quality care but also grant them access to sensitive and confidential information about patients. This access places students in a position of trust, where they must handle information with the utmost privacy and respect. Furthermore, the practice of healthcare is governed by regulations and policies that students are expected to follow, reinforcing the importance of their professional conduct.

To ensure that the student is embodying professional qualities, various aspects of the student's conduct should be evaluated regularly. This includes the student's communication style, which should facilitate clear and respectful interactions with peers and patients. Additionally, the student's overall image—including both the student's demeanour and appearance—plays a vital role in how the student is perceived by others. Competence in the student's field is essential, as is maintaining appropriate behaviour and a positive attitude in both academic and clinical settings. Together, these factors contribute to the student's professionalism and the trust placed in the student by patients and colleagues alike.

Examples of unprofessional practices that students should avoid include arriving late to class and leaving early, which can disrupt the learning environment. Being unprepared for group sessions can hinder collaboration and negatively impact the performance of the entire team. Furthermore, fostering bad relationships with colleagues or mentors can create a toxic atmosphere and inhibit professional growth. Other unprofessional behaviours include disrupting class sessions, failing to attend scheduled classes, and engaging in dishonest practices such as cheating on exams. These actions not only reflect poorly on the individual but also undermine the integrity of the healthcare profession.

Health science students should demonstrate behaviours and practices that foster self-development and professional development. First, punctuality and discipline are crucial aspects of character, as they indicate responsibility to oneself and others. These attributes facilitate efficient operations and a proper, timely flow of patients. In addition, integrity is important, as it ensures that patients and nurses are told the truth to promote trust and efficient delivery of healthcare services (Epstein 2002). Furthermore, patients' self-determination and confidentiality should always be honoured because they are the key principles of patient-centeredness. This respect recognizes patients as rational beings capable of making decisions regarding their health. In addition, grooming, dress, and neatness are important, as they show that the individual is credible and committed to providing proper patient care. Effective interpersonal skills are also crucial for the profession. The principles of active listening and the use of verbal and especially written language contribute to the effectiveness of cooperation and patient interactions, ultimately resulting in improved health outcomes (Levinson et al. 2010; Mobeireek et al. 1996).

For example, developing a friendly attitude will help put patients at ease when coming to the clinic or hospital. As important as artistry is, teamwork and collaboration in healthcare facilities are crucial for obtaining the best results. Self-development is also important, as seeking assistance when it is required shows respect and willingness to adopt new knowledge. In addition, one attribute that healthcare students must develop is patience. Patients with complicated diseases and complex communities of patients necessitate patience and compassion. Finally, perseverance is essential in gaining and retaining relevant knowledge and skills that are indispensable for professional proficiency. Thus, healthcare students can and should practice the behaviours described above to guarantee further medical development.

Finally, several obstacles can impede the journey to becoming a professional student. Poor training during either pre- or postgraduate education can leave students ill prepared for the demands of the profession. Unethical behaviour, student arrogance, a lack of faith in oneself or the profession, and work pressures are further challenges to professionalism. Additionally, exposure to negative community practices and friendships that encourage unprofessional behaviour can damage a student's ability to succeed. A lack of knowledge, failure to apply regulations such as codes of ethics and conduct, and a weak institutional and organizational system can all hinder the achievement of professionalism in the healthcare field. Figure 2.4 illustrates the professional behaviour of healthcare students.

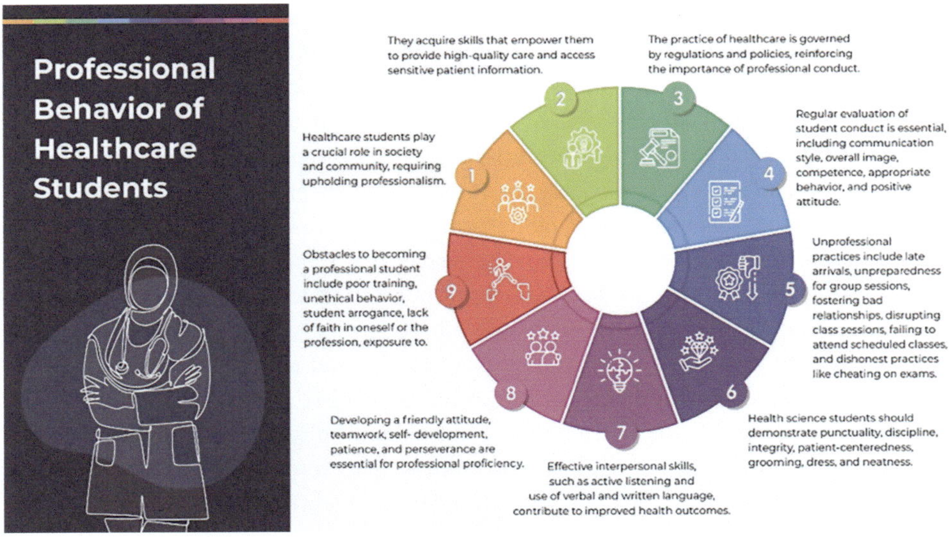

Fig. 2.4 Professional behaviour of healthcare students

2.10 Summary

A robust professional identity is foundational to a successful and ethical healthcare career. It is more than a mere collection of skills; it is the embodiment of values and behaviours that guide practitioners in their complex roles. By fostering a strong sense of respect, integrity, competence, teamwork, altruism, and advocacy, healthcare students lay the groundwork for a fulfilling career dedicated to patient well-being. The integration of Islamic ethics provides a moral compass, aligning with the core principles of professional identity and enriching the decision-making process. This framework emphasizes the importance of human dignity, justice, beneficence, nonmaleficence, and patient autonomy, fostering a compassionate and patient-centred approach to care. Cultivating a strong professional identity requires deliberate effort. Prioritizing professional demeanour, engaging in lifelong learning, and developing a patient-centred approach are essential. Furthermore, effective teamwork, ethical decision-making, and a commitment to service are indispensable. By embracing these values and behaviours, healthcare students can become exemplary professionals who not only deliver high-quality care but also contribute to a positive and ethical healthcare environment. This transformation is essential for addressing the complex challenges facing the healthcare industry and ensuring the well-being of patients and communities.

References

Adkoli BV, Al-Umran KU, Al-Sheikh M, Deepak KK, Al-Rubaish AM. Medical students' perception of professionalism: a qualitative study from Saudi Arabia. Med Teach. 2011;33:840–5.

Ali AIBM, Chamsi-Pasha H. Contemporary bioethics: Islamic perspective. Cham: Springer; 2015.

AlKhater SA. Perception of Saudi undergraduate students towards professionalism in medicine. Sultan Qaboos Univ Med J. 2021;21:378–85.

American Board of Medical Specialties Board of Directors. ABMS definition of medical professionalism (long form). 2012.

Arawi T. The ethics of the Muslim physician and the legacy of Muhammad. J Islam Med Assoc N Am. 2011;43:35–8.

Athar S, Fadel HE, Ahmed WD, Haque M, Nagamia HF, Hathout H, Amine ARC, Khan FA, Shanawani H. Islamic medical ethics: the IMANA perspective. JK Pract. 2005;12:231–7.

Beauchamp T, Childress J. Principles of biomedical ethics: marking its fortieth anniversary. Am J Bioeth. 2019;19:9–12.

Cruess SR, Cruess RL. Professionalism and medicine's social contract. Focus Health Prof Educ. 2014;16:4–19.

Epstein RM, Hundert EM. Defining and assessing professional competence. Journal of the American Medical Association (JAMA), 2002;287(2):226–235. https://doi.org/10.1001/jama.287.2.226

Glicken AD, Merenstein GB. Addressing the hidden curriculum: understanding educator professionalism. Med Teach. 2007;29:54–7.

Hedayat KM, Pirzadeh R. Issues in Islamic biomedical ethics: a primer for the pediatrician. Pediatrics. 2001;108:965–71.

Hussein GMA, Kaabba AFAI. Professionalism and ethics handbook for residents. Riyadh: Saudi Commission for Health Specialties; 2015.

Kasule OH. Biomedical ethics: an Islamic formulation. J Islam Med Assoc N Am. 2010;42:38–40.

Levinson W, Lesser CS, Epstein RM. Developing physician communication skills for patient-centered care. Health Aff. 2010;29:1310–8.

Mobeireek A, Al-Kassimi FA, Al-Majid SA, Al-Shimemry A. Communication with the seriously ill: physicians' attitudes in Saudi Arabia. J Med Ethics. 1996;22:282–5.

Padela AI. Islamic medical ethics: a primer. Bioethics. 2007;21:169–78.

How Medical and Health Science Students Think and Act as Champions

3

Khalid A. Bin Abdulrahman, Hassan Darami, and Sufyan Akram

Learning Objectives

1. *Understand the role of healthcare students as champions.*

   Explore how medical and health science students advocate for patient-centered care, ethical practices, and systemic improvements in healthcare delivery.
2. *Develop core competencies for effective healthcare practice.*

   Learn to integrate technical skills, critical thinking, and empathetic communication to improve patient outcomes and address diverse healthcare challenges.
3. *Apply ethical and reflective practices in professional growth.*

   Demonstrate the ability to navigate ethical dilemmas, promote equity in healthcare, and engage in reflective learning to enhance self-awareness and resilience in clinical settings.

K. A. Bin Abdulrahman (✉)
Department of Medical Education, College of Medicine, Imam Mohammad Ibn Saud Islamic University (IMSIU), Riyadh, Saudi Arabia
e-mail: kab@imamu.edu.sa

H. Darami
Department of Obstetrics & Gynecology and Medical Education, College of Medicine, Imam Mohammad Ibn Saud Islamic University (IMSIU), Riyadh, Saudi Arabia
e-mail: hwdarami@imamu.edu.sa

S. Akram
School of Medicine and Health, Charles Darwin University, Darwin, Australia
e-mail: sufyan.akram@cdu.edu.au

K. A. Bin Abdulrahman, H. Darami (eds.), *Essential Learning Skills for Health Professions Students*, https://doi.org/10.1007/978-981-96-5670-7_3

3.1 Introduction

Medical and health science students play central roles in the process of shaping the future of healthcare. As emerging professionals, these students are often personified by their pursuit of knowledge, skills, and attitudes. Empathy and a commitment to service represent the foundation of their ability to become ethical professionals. The unique learning landscape that characterizes the field of medicine and healthcare, which requires students to balance theoretical learning with practical application, cultivates critical thinking and a proactive approach to problem-solving. In many ways, these students are not merely learners but also advocates and champions who seek to promote better health outcomes in the wider community. This chapter explores the ways in which medical and health science students think and act as champions, particularly with respect to the following key areas: their knowledge and skills, including communication, their role in patient advocacy, and their commitment to leadership and ethical practice.

3.2 The Acquisition of Knowledge and Skills

One of the most significant ways in which medical and health science students act as champions is by embracing a scientific mindset. The education of such students is grounded in evidence-based practice (EBP), which emphasizes the use of the best available research and clinical expertise in the context of decision-making. This scientific approach fosters critical thinking, thereby enabling students to analyze complex data, synthesize information, and apply the knowledge they thus obtain to clinical settings. They are trained to question assumptions, identify gaps in knowledge, and approach problems methodically. This training lays a foundation for lifelong learning, which is an essential quality as medicine continues to evolve rapidly. New therapies, equipment, and approaches are being developed with increasing frequency. Hence, the ability to keep pace with the most recent trends in efforts to improve health outcomes is crucial. Sequential but autonomous learning, including continuing education, is essential in medicine. Smith (2019) rightly claimed that this receptiveness to formal learning, alongside the notion of self-learning, represents the foundation of lifelong learning in the context of healthcare.

Technical competencies are also crucial in this context. For example, when medical students are presented with a clinical case, they are encouraged to formulate differential diagnoses, rule out various possibilities systematically, and base their final decisions on the most up-to-date scientific evidence. This process not only enhances their diagnostic ability but also helps improve patient outcomes. The rigorous training in research methodology that these students undergo equips them to critically evaluate emerging studies and integrate new knowledge into their own practice, positioning them as champions of innovation and drivers of continuous improvement in healthcare. However, technical skills involve more than merely the set of clinical procedures that a professional normally performs. These skills require additional training, ethical practice, and the implementation of the knowledge acquired in this context; thus, medical and health science students must develop critical thinking and problem-solving competencies that extend beyond their core clinical competencies.

3.3 Effective Communication

The need for efficient communication among medical and health science students who aspire to be champions in this field can never be overemphasized. Communication between healthcare providers and patients is pivotal with respect to the delivery of high-quality care. Studies have consistently reported that good communication improves patient outcomes by increasing patients' satisfaction and adherence to treatment plans as well as by reducing the likelihood of misunderstandings and errors. One study, which was conducted by Stewart et al. (2000), revealed that "patients who experience better communication with their physicians have better recovery rates and fewer emotional problems." Effective communication can facilitate the establishment of trust, which is an essential component of the therapeutic relationship, and help promote shared decision-making, thus enabling patients to play an active role in decisions concerning their healthcare (Epstein et al. 2005).

For medical students, the ability to communicate effectively with patients is a core competency that must be developed during training. Medical students learn how to communicate complex medical information in a way that is both understandable and empathetic, including by tailoring their language to the patient's level of health literacy. This skill is particularly important in culturally diverse settings, in which language barriers, cultural differences, and varying levels of education can pose significant challenges with regard to communication.

Effective communication in medicine extends beyond the mere exchange of information; rather, it also involves empathy, emotional intelligence, cultural sensitivity, and active listening. Empathy, which refers to the ability to understand and share the feelings of others, is a critical component of the patient–physician relationship. Empathetic communication improves patient satisfaction and leads to better patient outcomes by reducing anxiety, fostering trust, and encouraging patients to be more open with respect to their symptoms and concerns (Mercer and Reynolds 2002).

According to Greenwood et al. (2020), understanding communication skills is essential with regard to efforts to increase patient compliance and improve health outcomes. Courses that address these areas can help students increase their sensitivity and attentiveness to patient requirements. Moreover, Greenwood et al. (2020) investigated active listening practices that healthcare providers can use to pay careful attention to patients' questions or concerns as well as to ensure that patients feel that they are engaged in a partnership with the healthcare providers who treat them. Communication skills also include cultural sensitivity, which enables students to treat patients' diseases in a culturally sensitive manner while simultaneously recognizing that different cultures are characterized by different perceptions of disease diagnosis and treatment as well as other practices.

3.4 Commitment to Patient Care

Perhaps, the most important factor that defines a champion in the context of healthcare is patient care. The delivery of such care requires healthcare providers to recognize and support patients' choices, which are crucial in the process of providing sensitive care and support to patients. Jones et al. (2018) claimed that, in addition to delivering clinical care to patients, understanding patients' needs can help promote positive health outcomes for patients. Patient-centered care addresses not only the physical nature of contact with patients. It also involves evaluations of the biological, psychological, social, and spiritual aspects of patients as well as their symptoms and illnesses.

As mentioned, while a scientific mindset is crucial in this context, medical and health science students must also exhibit compassion and empathy; these qualities are central to their role as patient advocates. As champions of patient-centered care, these students are trained to view patients holistically, including by considering not only their physical health but also their emotional, social, and psychological well-being. Such a focus on communication skills, cultural competency, and ethical decision-making is integral to the ability of these students to develop into compassionate professionals.

In clinical settings, students often serve as intermediaries between patients and the healthcare system, including by advocating for their patients' rights and ensuring that patients' voices are heard. In various contexts, such as navigating complex treatment plans, communicating diagnoses, or managing end-of-life care for patients, students are taught to prioritize the autonomy and dignity of their patients. This advocacy is especially important with respect to underserved populations, in which context students often play various roles in community outreach programs, health education, and preventive care. By serving as champions of health equity, students work to reduce disparities and improve access to healthcare among vulnerable populations.

Another aspect of this commitment to patient care pertains to students' obligations with regard to quality improvement and, thus, self-review. These obligations are essential with respect to students' personal and professional development. These reflective practices allow students to evaluate their clinical skills, communication abilities, and ethical decision-making processes. Such self-assessments can help students identify areas for improvement, thereby promoting continuous learning and the development of a growth mindset, which represents an essential quality of champions that enables them to adapt to the evolving field of healthcare. This introspection can help students obtain a deeper understanding of patient-centered care by enabling students to learn to recognize and manage their biases and reactions. Such awareness is vital with regard to students' efforts to maintain a high standard of care and establish strong patient–provider relationships.

Additionally, working within diverse medical and healthcare teams requires interdisciplinary collaboration. Such interdisciplinary collaboration is crucial with regard to the task of promoting patient-centered, integrated care, which can ultimately improve public health. Moreover, patient care involves adherence to professional and ethical standards even in the most difficult situations. This process facilitates the establishment of a foundation of integrity, professionalism, and trust in the context of patient care. When students adhere to ethical guidelines, they can make sound decisions, exhibit empathy, and ensure respect for diverse values and backgrounds. Such a commitment to ethical practice is essential with respect to the tasks of building public trust and ensuring high-quality, compassionate care. Further details regarding this point are provided in the following section.

Finally, it is essential for medical and health science students to be active advocates for the provision and enhancement of patient care at both the micro- and macrolevels. Such advocacy includes presenting evidence-based recommendations to interprofessional healthcare teams and collaborating with such teams to facilitate necessary changes. For example, students may engage in quality improvement initiatives, research patient care processes, and participate in policy-making activities pertaining to healthcare delivery. By engaging in these efforts, students can contribute meaningfully to the task of improving healthcare systems worldwide.

3.5 Ethical Decision-Making

A key aspect of professional practice in healthcare is ethical decision-making. Medical and health science students must be prepared to navigate complex ethical challenges while adhering to the principles of autonomy, beneficence, nonmaleficence, and justice, as highlighted by Beauchamp and Childress (2019). These principles guide healthcare providers' efforts to protect patients' interests while respecting patients' rights and dignity.

Students must be ready to confront ethical dilemmas by engaging in rational and fair decision-making, including by understanding the ethical implications of their actions and being able to explain these implications to relevant stakeholders. Students' ethical competence can be enhanced through case presentations and simulations, which provide students with the independence they need to practice solving real-world ethical challenges while simultaneously fostering strong relationships with their patients and colleagues.

Patient autonomy is central to ethical practice. Students must respect patients' right to make informed decisions regarding their treatment, including by understanding and communicating patients' health status, management options, and relevant potential outcomes. Integrating the principle of autonomy with those of beneficence and nonmaleficence can help ensure that compassionate and patient-centered care is delivered.

Ethical decision-making also involves managing conflicts of interest. Medical students are expected to make impartial decisions, including by acknowledging and addressing any personal, financial, or professional conflicts that could compromise patient care. Training in ethics should cover ways of managing conflicts of interest and methods that can be used to maintain professionalism. Justice, which is another fundamental ethical principle, mandates that all patients should be treated in an equitable manner, regardless of social status, race, or other factors. Students should serve as advocates for health equity, including by participating in initiatives aimed at empowering underserved populations and challenging biases in healthcare. Transparency and accountability are also crucial with respect to ethical decision-making. Medical students should exhibit openness in their actions and clearly communicate decisions to patients, families, and peers. Ethical education should emphasize recording decisions, seeking second opinions when necessary, and admitting one's mistakes. Peer and mentor discussions concerning ethical issues can encourage students to adopt diverse perspectives, thereby reinforcing ethical standards within the healthcare community.

In summary, ethical decision-making is a collaborative process that can be enriched by communal norms and values, which collectively strengthen healthcare students' commitment to high ethical standards in practice.

3.6 Leadership

The terms "student leaders" and "student champions" are sometimes used interchangeably, but they have distinct meanings that depend on the context at hand. Details concerning the differences between these terms are provided here. Student leaders are individuals who occupy formal leadership positions, often within student organizations, committees, or groups. They are responsible for guiding and managing their peers, for organizing activities, and occasionally for representing the institutions or groups with which they are associated. The focus of such student leaders is often on governance, coordination, and the long-term success of a team or organization. Leadership involves setting directions, making decisions, and delegating tasks. Student champions, on the other hand, are advocates or role models who passionately promote specific causes, innovations, or ideas. They are less concerned with formal leadership roles than student leaders and more concerned with specific issues or projects about which they care deeply. Thus, the focus of such student champions is on advocacy, inspiration, and efforts to promote change. They may not hold official titles, but they rally support and encourage others to participate in initiatives pertaining to their chosen cause (e.g., mental health awareness, sustainability in medical practices, or patient care quality). Champions are informal leaders, and beginning at an early point in their education, they become aware of the importance of interprofessional collaboration, teamwork, and ethical leadership in healthcare settings. As future physicians, nurses, or allied health professionals, these champions are encouraged to develop strong leadership skills, which are essential for their efforts to guide teams, manage healthcare resources, and advocate for systemic change. Champions thus tend to be persuasive, enthusiastic, and driven by personal conviction.

Furthermore, as future healthcare professionals, students are increasingly expected to serve as advocates for broader societal issues, including climate change, healthcare policy reform, and public health crises such as pandemics and climate change. In so doing, they act as champions with respect to the health of not only individual patients but also entire populations. Students' involvement in global health initiatives, policy advocacy, and community health projects thus reflects a deep commitment to the tasks of improving healthcare systems and addressing the social determinants of health.

3.7 Reflecting on Personal Experiences

Reflective learning is a vital tool with respect to the professional growth of medical and health science students; namely, it can help students develop self-awareness and set meaningful personal and professional goals. As noted by Schön (2017), reflection in the context of professional practice involves processing knowledge that one has acquired by performing various tasks, thus allowing students to analyze their clinical experiences, their interactions with patients, and the outcomes of their actions. Such reflective critique can help students identify areas for improvement and enhance their future practice.

Reflective practice also promotes resilience, as it helps students manage the emotional and ethical challenges that are inherent to patient care. Ultimately, reflection equips students to deliver high-quality, compassionate care and to adapt to the evolving demands of healthcare.

Reflection can be enriched through collaborative learning, such as peer discussions and mentorship programs, which provide students with valuable feedback and broaden their perspectives on practice. Reflective journals and portfolios serve as effective tools that students can use to record their learning journeys, track their progress, and celebrate their achievements. By embedding reflection into their practices, medical and health science students can strengthen their clinical competencies and obtain a deeper understanding of their professional roles and responsibilities.

3.8 A Ten-step Plan for the Acquisition of the Characteristics of a Student Champion

Becoming a student champion requires a combination of passion, advocacy, leadership, and dedication to a specific cause or issue about which one cares deeply. Unlike those who play formal leadership roles, student champions are often recognized for their influence, impact, and commitment to the task of driving change within their communities. Table 3.1 summarizes the ten steps involved in the process of becoming a champion. Let us refer to these steps as a champion's toolkit, as also shown Fig. 3.1.

Another useful tip in this context is to keep track of one's activities. This goal can be achieved by maintaining a digital progress tracker. In addition, quantitative metrics (e.g., event participation or social media engagement) and qualitative data (e.g., feedback and testimonials) can be collected. Finally, individuals' achievements can be documented, and their success can be celebrated and shared.

Table 3.1 The ten-step plan for the acquisition of the characteristics of a student champion

Step	Action
1	Identify a cause or issue you are passionate about
2	Develop a clear vision and goals related to the chosen cause
3	Gain knowledge and understanding about the cause through research and learning
4	Build technical skills and competencies necessary to advocate effectively
5	Develop effective communication skills to convey your message and inspire others
6	Collaborate with peers and interdisciplinary teams to amplify your impact
7	Engage in advocacy efforts and actively participate in initiatives or events
8	Monitor and track your activities, progress, and outcomes to measure impact
9	Collect feedback and testimonials to refine your approach and strategies
10	Celebrate and share your achievements to inspire and motivate others to join your efforts

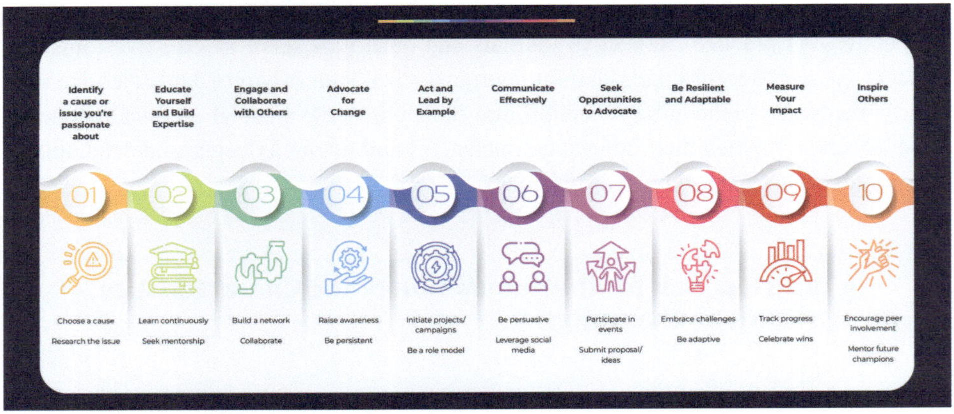

Fig. 3.1 A ten-step plan for the acquisition of the characteristics of a student champion

3.9 Summary

Medical and health science students respond to the situations that they face and serve as champions on the basis of the knowledge and skills that they have acquired as well as their professionalism, communication, and ethical understanding. These competencies enable students to acquire new skills and knowledge continuously, thereby allowing them to adapt effectively to advancements in their field as well as to enhance the quality of patient care. The principles that underlie a patient-centered care environment ensure that patient welfare remains a top priority in this context. Communication and collaboration are foundational values that foster trust, particularly in the context of technological innovation, whereas ethical decision-making supports the integrity of the healthcare profession. Reflective practice supports students' professional growth by strengthening their resilience and increasing their capacity to manage stress. Collectively, these elements empower medical and health science students to excel in terms of their professional responsibilities, thereby ultimately improving the quality, effectiveness, and complementary value of the healthcare services that they provide to patients.

References

Beauchamp TL, Childress JF. Principles of biomedical ethics. Oxford: Oxford University Press; 2019.

Epstein RM, Alper BS, Quill TE. Communicating evidence for participatory decision-making. JAMA. 2005;293:1371–8.

Greenwood RM, Maddox K, Smith JL. Effective communication in healthcare: a guide for practitioners. Springer; Cham, Switzerland, 2020.

Jones J, Hunter D, Murphy K. Health care providers in the next decade: champions for patients in a changing health care system. J Healthc Manag. 2018;63:380–93.

Mercer SW, Reynolds WJ. Empathy and quality of care. Br J Gen Pract. 2002;52(Suppl):S9–S12.

Schön DA. The reflective practitioner: how professionals think in action. New York: Routledge; 2017.

Smith M. Lifelong learning in medicine and healthcare: principles and practices. Springer; Cham, Switzerland, 2019.

Stewart M, Judith B, Brown AD, McWhinney IR, Julian Oates W, Weston W, Jordan J. The impact of patient-centered care on outcomes. J Fam Pract. 2000;49:796–804.

Getting the Most Out of New Trends in Health Profession Education

4

Khalid A. Bin Abdulrahman

Learning Objectives

1. Understand key innovations in health profession education.
   - Identify modern educational approaches, including PBL, TBL, simulation-based learning, and advanced assessment tools like OSCEs and electronic portfolios.
2. Enhance learning through engagement and innovation.
   - Explore strategies for utilizing innovative learning methods, engaging with scholarly resources, and participating in professional development.
3. Prepare for future careers in healthcare.
   - Recognize the importance of interdisciplinary teamwork, continuous improvement, and resource utilization to succeed in healthcare education and practice.

4.1 Introduction

The field of health profession education is continuously developing, integrating groundbreaking methods to improve learning outcomes. As medical and health science learners navigate these dynamic settings, it is important for them to comprehend and adapt to such new trends to be successful in their careers. For example, research has revealed that the practice of medicine is increasingly dependent on teams of professionals addressing

K. A. Bin Abdulrahman (✉)
Department of Medical Education, College of Medicine, Imam Mohammad Ibn Saud Islamic University (IMSIU), Riyadh, Saudi Arabia
e-mail: kab@imamu.edu.sa

K. A. Bin Abdulrahman, H. Darami (eds.), *Essential Learning Skills for Health Professions Students*, https://doi.org/10.1007/978-981-96-5670-7_4

multifaceted cases and patients with diverse chronic conditions. This chapter suggests how learners can maximize their learning experience and benefit the most from the existing trends in health profession education.

4.2 Exploring the Most Common Trends in Learning and Teaching in Healthcare Education

Today, adjustments in political and economic conditions, developments in science and technology, and advancements in epidemiology and sociology have influenced the transformation of health and medical education systems. Research has revealed that as a result of the nature of medical education, new teaching approaches and their employment in teaching-learning are crucial (Abianeh et al. 2022). The quality of medical services relies on medical education, and emerging trends play a crucial role in shaping the delivery of care. Therefore, the most common trends in learning and teaching in healthcare education include the following:

4.2.1 New Curricula

Indications that there is a need to focus on medical education are not new. Research shows that the traditional undergraduate medical curriculum has been subject to intense criticism throughout the last few periods for being disjointed and burdensome and forcing learners to learn by rote and attain knowledge passively rather than through inquisitiveness and exploration (Mittal and Medhi 2022). Moreover, the need to implement considerable changes in the content of undergraduate medical curricula and teaching and evaluation approaches has long been felt. However, there have been recent developments in medical education that have led to the integration of diverse new ideas into healthcare fields. In response to the recent advancements in healthcare, educational institutions are currently reviewing curricula with the aim of integrating cutting-edge knowledge and skills (Mittal and Medhi 2022). New curricula mostly rely on integrated learning, where basic and clinical sciences are taught concurrently. This strategy helps learners comprehend the relevance of foundational knowledge in clinical practice.

4.2.2 Problem-Based Learning (PBL)

PBL is a teaching method whereby learners actively participate in real-world and personally meaningful projects. Research describes PBL as a student-centred pedagogy in which learning arises through the active resolution of real-world, open-ended issues (Ghani et al. 2021). This stands in contrast to some traditional educational approaches in which educators present facts and ideas directly to learners. It places learners in the role of active problem-solvers, supporting them in engaging deeply with the material. This approach nurtures critical thinking, self-directed learning, and the ability to utilize knowledge in practical scenarios. In PBL, learners basically work in small groups, with every member contributing unique ideas and gaining proficiency. This collaborative setting supports peer learning and improves communication skills among learners.

The groups are usually presented with a multifaceted, real-world issue that lacks a clear explanation. Through guided inquiry, learners identify what they understand, what they want to learn, and how to bridge this gap (Ghani et al. 2021). This process comprises researching, hypothesizing, testing solutions, and reflecting on results. Table 4.1 summarizes the Maastricht seven-jump process for PBL.

4.2.3 Task-Based Learning (TBL)

TBL is an educational strategy that emphasizes tasks indispensable to professional practice. While using TBL, learners are given specific projects to complete, allowing them to develop practical skills and capabilities that are directly applicable to their future careers. This approach stresses hands-on experience and active learning, relating theoretical knowledge to its practical application. Research shows that the need for improved professional capabilities in medical scholars has necessitated a transformation in the curricula used by medical institutes in recent years (Shenoy et al. 2022). For example, units that offer reactive answers rather than premeditated responses, which require critical thinking and conversant decision-making skills, are preferred in preclinical learning. Preclinical education is the initial stage in a medical curriculum that comprises the fundamental sciences that offer the basis for subsequent clinical practice.

The major problem for instructors has been to make preclinical education more connected to the roles of healthcare professionals. Research has shown that the early inclusion

Table 4.1 Summary of the Maastricht seven-jump process for problem-based learning (PBL)

Step	Description
1. Clarify terms	Identify and clarify any unclear terms or concepts in the problem
2. Define the problem	Agree on a clear and concise statement of the problem to be addressed
3. Brainstorm	List all possible explanations, ideas, or hypotheses about the problem
4. Structure & organize	Group related ideas, rank hypotheses, and create a framework for investigation
5. Formulate learning objectives	Define specific questions or objectives for further research and study
6. Independent study	Research the learning objectives independently, using various resources
7. Discuss & synthesize	Share findings, discuss solutions, and apply new knowledge to the problem

of clinical applications in the curricula in medical courses forces preclinical courses to address the most important topics in medical education (Shenoy et al. 2022). Through preclinical task-based learning (TBL), early clinical exposures have been made more participatory, encompassing different approaches during small-group training meetings. Today, consistent patient encounters can be easily integrated into the clinical undergraduate education, and TBL has been utilized and acknowledged as a beneficial tool throughout the clinical clerkship period in many medical institutes. Table 4.2 summarizes the comparison of problem-based learning and task-based learning.

4.2.4 Simulation-Based Learning

The idea of simulation-based learning has existed in healthcare education for a long time. However, simulation-based learning has been adopted by many healthcare institutions at various points to enhance real-world skills, preparedness, and confidence, thereby ensuring patient well-being and improved real-world patient care. Research describes simulation-based education as including the knowledge, behaviours, and skills obtained by healthcare experts that improve patient-centric care (Saleem and Khan 2023). As a result of legal and ethical concerns, the traditional ways of learning that involved cadavers, animals' studies, and patients are becoming less tolerated. Simulation provides learners and educators with a chance to reconstruct specific cases that cannot otherwise be studied in a controlled learning environment. These cases are not useful for individual study but can be utilized for learning in teams and organizations.

Healthcare education institutions across the world are adopting simulation as a learning tool to help learners develop skills and managerial strategies by engaging with realistic situational encounters without affecting patient safety. Such engagement in simulations in medical education is intended to imitate the real world and offer new healthcare learners the chance to practice skills and diagnostic strategies on 'computer-guided models in a professional way' (Saleem and Khan 2023). Moreover, simulation-based learning has led healthcare experts to work interprofessionally towards the shared goal of patient-focused care.

Virtual reality (VR) and augmented reality (AR) technologies have further enhanced simulation-based learning by immersing learners in detailed, lifelike settings where they can practice procedures and clinical decision-making. VR can transport learners to a fully digital environment, whereas AR overlays digital data onto the real world, enhancing the learning experience with important information. Research shows that such approaches are especially vital for training in emergency practices and multifaceted medical interventions, where practicing in real-world conditions might be impossible or too risky (Tene et al. 2024). For example, learners can participate in a simulated cardiac arrest case, practising CPR and defibrillation on a mannequin, which offers real-time feedback on their performance. Surgical simulation allows learners to develop and improve their techniques in the absence of the pressure and consequences of operating on live patients.

Table 4.2 Comparison of problem-based learning and task-based learning

Aspect	Problem-based learning (PBL)	Task-based learning (TBL)
Definition	PBL is a student-centred approach where learners solve real-world problems to acquire knowledge and skills	TBL focuses on completing meaningful tasks that replicate real-life activities to learn a language or subject
Primary goal	Develop critical thinking, problem-solving skills, and deep understanding of concepts	Enhance practical skills, fluency, and specific task-related competencies
Nature of activity	Learners work on open-ended, complex problems without predefined solutions	Learners engage in completing structured tasks with clear objectives and outcomes
Instructional approach	Guided discovery with minimal direct teaching; teachers act as facilitators	Direct or semi-guided instruction with specific task completion as the focus; teachers may provide feedback
Collaboration	Collaborative group work is central, often involving group discussions and shared responsibilities	Collaboration may or may not be required, depending on the task's design
Content focus	Interdisciplinary, integrating knowledge from various fields to solve the problem	Task-specific, focusing on practical application and contextual language or skill use
Assessment	Often formative, based on group performance, process evaluation, and solution quality	Usually performance-based, focusing on task completion and the effectiveness of the final output
Learner's role	Active problem-solvers, responsible for identifying learning gaps and seeking solutions	Active task performers, applying knowledge to achieve specific goals
Teacher's role	Facilitator and guide, helping students explore and reflect on their learning process	Instructor or coach, providing support, feedback, and sometimes explicit instruction during tasks
Examples	Diagnosing and proposing solutions for a public health issue, designing an engineering project	Writing an email, organizing a trip, conducting a presentation, or role-playing a real-world scenario
Strengths	Develops lifelong learning skills, promotes deeper understanding, and fosters collaboration	Improves task-specific skills, encourages real-world application, and enhances practical communication abilities
Challenges	Time-intensive, requires skilled facilitation, and may overwhelm learners without proper scaffolding	May oversimplify concepts, risk of focusing more on task completion than underlying understanding

Key Differences

- *Purpose*: PBL emphasizes problem-solving and conceptual understanding, while TBL emphasizes practical application and task fluency
- *Structure*: PBL is typically more open-ended and exploratory, whereas TBL has more defined objectives and outcomes
- *Collaboration*: Collaboration is more integral to PBL, while TBL can be both individual and group based

Both approaches are highly effective in fostering active learning, and their use depends on the goals of the educational program and the learners' needs

4.2.5 New Assessment Tools

Assessment methods are a recent field that has undergone the greatest transformation in terms of progress with regard to educational technology. Research shows that most of the assessment methods used in medical education are 'paper-written, oral, or practical texts' (Park et al. 2021). The greatest challenge associated with written tests involves the difficulty with offering enough feedback to learners as a result of the structural influence of the overwhelmingly smaller number of assessors compared with the number of learners. However, innovative tools are emerging that are revolutionizing how learners' knowledge, skills, and behaviours are assessed and providing an exhaustive means of determining their readiness for professional practice. For example, tools such as objective structured clinical examinations (OSCEs), formative assessments, and electronic portfolios have been useful in medical education.

Research has identified OSCEs as the most commonly used assessment tool for evaluating practical skills among medical students (Giri and Stewart 2023). In an OSCE, learners rotate through a series of stations where they carry out clinical inspections, perform procedures, and take medical histories. Each station is often standardized and utilizes trained actors or high-fidelity mannequins, ensuring that the assessment is consistent. OSCEs offer objective, structured, and direct assessments of clinical competencies, allowing for thorough feedback on each learner's performance.

Formative assessments are meant to offer consistent feedback during the learning process. Research shows that 'feedback on formative and summative evaluations' is designed to bridge detected gaps in learning but remains a passive procedure, and its success relies on learner follow-through (Lakhtakia et al. 2022). The finest exercise in evaluation suggests that passed the 'assessment of learning (AoL),' which is summative and defines the realization of results, 'assessment for learning (AfL)' through 'formative criticism and assessment as learning (AaL),' which is learner-centric, has been crucial for enhancing students' intellectual skills.

The electronic portfolio, also known as an e-portfolio, provides a dynamic way for learners to document and reflect on their learning experiences over time. These portfolios collect a range of evidence, such as written reflections, case studies, peer reviews, and procedural logs (Janssens et al. 2022). Continuous documentation helps learners track their progress, identify areas for improvement, and demonstrate their competencies to teachers and future employers.

These assessment tools ensure that the evaluations are not only comprehensive but also supportive of the learner's growth and development. By integrating continuous feedback and reflection into the learning process, these approaches help learners build the competence and confidence needed for effective professional practice.

4.2.6 Peer and Near-Peer Teaching and Assessment

Peer education is a broadly utilized teaching approach where learners educate their peers and junior learners. Research has identified a near-peer teacher (NPT) as an individual who is at least 'one-year elder to their near-peer learner (NPL) in the context of medical training' (Lucia and Wedemeyer 2021). The peer-to-peer method of teaching was initially introduced in 1988 by Whitman and Fife, who reported the use of peer education approaches in tertiary teaching settings. As early as the 1950s, undergraduate learners were active in instruction and laboratory support to save educational time and reduce lecture-based didactic learning. As it has gained acceptance over time, the benefits of peer education have been reinforced by 'subjective and objective evidence' (Lucia and Wedemeyer 2021). Students find that peer education advances their comprehension of subject topics and provides information at a suitable level.

The current NPTPs are designed to teach clinical skills in isolation instead of the approaches needed for OSCEs and the art of incorporating clinical skills (Lucia and Wedemeyer 2021). Explaining ideas to peers helps improve the educator's knowledge while offering the student a different perspective. This collaborative strategy also nurtures communication skills, critical thinking, and shared respect among learners. NPTPs help bridge the gap between theoretical skill and practical usage, as senior learners might share their recent experiences and practical understanding with juniors. Near-peer teaching helps junior learners relate more easily to ideas, seeing them through the eyes of somebody who has newly navigated these challenges (Lucia and Wedemeyer 2021). Senior learners can benefit from consolidating their knowledge and growing their leadership and mentoring skills.

4.3 Recognizing Student, Faculty, and Administrative Expectations

Recognizing the expectations of all stakeholders is important for enabling learners to thrive in their educational journeys. Research shows that positive stakeholder relationships are not just beneficial because they are critical to the achievements of any educational institution (Wilson and Brown 2019). It is similar to an art and science, which educational leaders must master to direct the tide of public opinion, ensure a supportive setting, and foster community goodwill. Therefore, to effectively navigate new trends in health profession education, understanding students, faculty, and administrative expectations is crucial.

4.3.1 Student Expectations

For learners to navigate new trends in health profession education, they should actively utilize innovative learning approaches comprising simulation-based learning and PBL. Remaining informed by engaging with scholarly sources, workshops, and conferences is important (Johnson and Stevens 2020). Students must accept new assessment strategies and take part in peer and near-peer teaching to advance their understanding and capabilities. Seeking ongoing feedback, collaborating with peers, and engaging with available resources, such as online platforms and virtual simulations, can further advance their learning. By connecting their hard work to faculty expectations and being proactive students, they can successfully acclimatize to and benefit from evolving educational methods.

4.3.2 Faculty Expectations

Faculty members must offer clear guidelines that support student-centred learning and promote open communication. Staying up to date with studies on learning methods and technological growth allows them to incorporate cutting-edge tools, such as VA, and new assessment tools, such as e-portfolios and OSCEs (Amerstorfer and von Münster-Kistner 2021). Participating in professional development opportunities and working together with co-workers across disciplines can improve their teaching approaches. By nurturing a supportive and interactive learning setting, offering timely feedback, and encouraging active student involvement, faculty can successfully familiarize themselves with and lead the implementation of such emerging educational strategies.

4.3.3 Administrative Expectations

Administrations can navigate new trends in health profession education by capitalizing on innovative technologies and resources, including digital learning platforms and high-fidelity simulations. Supporting faculty development through training programs ensures that teachers are prepared to execute innovative teaching approaches. Nurturing interdisciplinary teamwork and facilitating partnerships with healthcare organizations can improve practical learning opportunities for learners (Amerstorfer and von Münster-Kistner 2021). Administrators must emphasize establishing flexible, student-centred curricula and innovative approaches to assessment while ensuring that policies and infrastructure support such advancements. Regular assessment and adaptation of educational approaches based on feedback and evolving trends will help ensure a dynamic and functional learning environment.

4.4 Getting the Most Out of Educational Approaches

To improve their learning experience, learners should actively participate in the various educational techniques implemented in their programs by attending lectures and workshops, engaging in group discussions and practical sessions, and seeking clarification when necessary. Active involvement in discussion and group activities improves comprehension and knowledge retention (Smith 2021). Making use of the available resources, including virtual simulations, online learning platforms, and interactive tools, is important in modern health profession education. These resources are crucial because they offer more practice and reinforce learning.

Seeking feedback regularly from educators and peers is crucial because it helps learners identify areas that need improvement and develop their skills. Constructive feedback is important for continuous learning and growth. Moreover, developing critical thinking skills is crucial. Engaging in PBL and TBL helps learners develop their critical thinking skills. By addressing real-world issues and tasks, learners learn to examine, produce, and utilize knowledge in practical circumstances (Smith 2021). Interdisciplinary learning encourages teamwork across different healthcare workers. Learners should engage in interdisciplinary activities to gain a broader perspective and understand the significance of collaboration in healthcare.

In conclusion, for educational institutions to make the most of new trends in health profession education, learners must actively participate in the learning process, remain updated about the newest developments, and align their hard work with the expectations of faculty and administrators. By embracing new elements of curricula, such as TBL, PBL, simulation-based learning, innovative assessment tools, and peer teaching, learners can promote their learning experience, develop critical skills, and prepare themselves for the evolving healthcare landscape. Therefore, the keys to success in health profession education lie in active participation, continuous improvement, and the utilization of resources. As learners adapt to new trends and educational techniques, they will be better equipped to meet the demands of their future careers and contribute to the advancement of healthcare.

4.5 Summary

Health profession education is constantly evolving, incorporating new methodologies like problem-based learning, task-based learning, simulation-based learning, and innovative assessment tools like objective structured clinical examinations (OSCEs), formative assessments, and electronic portfolios. To succeed, learners must actively engage with new learning strategies, stay informed, engage with scholarly literature, and participate in professional development opportunities. Administrators can address emerging trends by using new technologies, promoting multidisciplinary collaboration, and creating adaptable courses.

References

Abianeh NA, Yazdani S, Heydari M, Farmad SA. Global perspectives on trends in health higher education. J Family Med Prim Care. 2022;11:4991–5003.

Amerstorfer CM, von Münster-Kistner CF. Student perceptions of academic engagement and student-teacher relationships in problem-based learning. Front Psychol. 2021;12:713057.

Ghani AS, Abdul AF, Rahim A, Yusoff MSB, Hadie SNH. Effective learning behavior in problem-based learning: a scoping review. Med Sci Educ. 2021;31:1199–211.

Giri J, Stewart C. Innovations in assessment in health professions education during the COVID-19 pandemic: a scoping review. Clin Teach. 2023;20:e13634.

Janssens O, Haerens L, Valcke M, Beeckman D, Pype P, Embo M. The role of ePortfolios in supporting learning in eight healthcare disciplines: a scoping review. Nurse Educ Pract. 2022;63:103418.

Johnson B, Stevens C. Student expectations in health professions education. Int J Health Prof Educ. 2020;12:145–62.

Lakhtakia R, Otaki F, Alsuwaidi L, Zary N. Assessment as learning in medical education: feasibility and perceived impact of student-generated formative assessments. JMIR Med Educ. 2022;8:e35820.

Lucia VC, Wedemeyer R. Evaluating effectiveness of faculty and near-peer delivered teaching and communication skills training. Med Sci Educ. 2021;31:1019–24.

Mittal N, Medhi B. New undergraduate medical education curriculum. Indian J Pharmacol. 2022;54:73–6.

Park J-C, Kwon H-JE, Chung CW. Innovative digital tools for new trends in teaching and assessment methods in medical and dental education. J Educ Eval Health Prof. 2021;18:13.

Saleem M, Khan Z. Healthcare simulation: an effective way of learning in health care. Pak J Med Sci. 2023;39:1185–90.

Shenoy R, Jain A, Bhagyalakshmi K, Shirali A, Shetty SB, Ramakrishna A. A task-based learning strategy in preclinical medical education. Adv Physiol Educ. 2022;46:192–9.

Smith A. Innovative approaches in health professions education. J Med Educ. 2021;45:87–102.

Tene T, López DFV, Aguirre PEV, Puente LMO, Gomez CV. Virtual reality and augmented reality in medical education: an umbrella review. Front Digit Health. 2024;6:1365345.

Wilson D, Brown K. Strategies for getting the most out of educational approaches in health professions. J Health Prof Adv. 2019;8:33–46.

Student Engagement and Active Learning in Health Profession Education

5

Khalid A. Bin Abdulrahman and Barbara Barzansky

Learning Objectives

1. Define and articulate the key components of student engagement in health profession education, including active learning and institutional partnerships.
2. Identify and evaluate strategies to foster active learning and student participation in institutional decision-making, curriculum evaluation, research, and community engagement.
3. Analyse common barriers to student engagement and propose institutional actions and cultural shifts necessary to overcome these challenges effectively.

5.1 Introduction

Students in health profession programs are on a lifelong journey that requires both the ability and willingness to continue to learn. This habit of learning should be encouraged and supported by the educational process so that learners are prepared for their future away from a structured educational environment. Such preparation includes instilling both the desire to continue to learn and the skills to do so. Therefore, teachers should not only address students' immediate learning needs but also help them accept responsibility for their continued learning. One way to accomplish this objective is to create an environment that allows students to be engaged with how they learn and how they partner with their learning environment to develop skills and attitudes that contribute to lifelong learning.

K. A. Bin Abdulrahman (✉)
Department of Medical Education, College of Medicine, Imam Mohammad Ibn Saud Islamic University (IMSIU), Riyadh, Saudi Arabia
e-mail: kab@imamu.edu.sa

B. Barzansky
American Medical Association, Chicago, IL, USA
e-mail: barbara.barzansky@ama-assn.org

K. A. Bin Abdulrahman, H. Darami (eds.), *Essential Learning Skills for Health Professions Students*, https://doi.org/10.1007/978-981-96-5670-7_5

The availability of opportunities for engagement is broadly considered an important component of health profession education quality (Kassab et al. 2023).

5.2 The Components of Student Engagement

Kassab et al. (2023) described two components of student engagement: (1) students' engagement in their own learning and (2) students' engagement in their educational environment through partnerships. This definition encompasses both the learner as an individual and the learner as an active member of and participant in the activities of an educational institution, which requires both that students are willing to be engaged and that the organizational environment is welcoming and supportive of their participation.

5.3 Student Engagement as Active Learners

Active learning is an example of students' engagement in and responsibility for their own learning. Active learning is most simply described as a process in which students engage rather than just an instructional method (Gavarkovs et al. 2024). This concrete definitional approach removes the limits on the type of engagement and focuses on what and how the learner thinks (cognitive engagement) or does (behavioural engagement). In active learning, students are not merely passive recipients of knowledge but also have the opportunity and ability to identify their learning needs and to actively seek information to meet them. We illustrate this definition using the example of a medical microbiology course in a health profession education program. In this course, a traditional lecture-based teaching method is compared with a learning approach that stresses student responsibility and active participation.

Evidence has shown that active learning processes "work" (Michael 2006) in that they can produce better performance outcomes and more and deeper learning and retention than passive learning methods. This is because one of the main advantages of active learning is improved comprehension and knowledge retention (Lombardi et al. 2021). The incorporation of active learning techniques and methods such as problem-solving tasks, active discussions, and practical assignments provides the learner with a meaningful way of interacting with and processing information rather than passively receiving it, which ensures that students internalize their understanding of the content and makes it easier to remember and apply. This kind of engagement also improves student memory and enables them to apply such knowledge to their profession in real-life situations. Table 5.1 provides a comparison of traditional lecture-based and active learning instructional processes.

Table 5.1 A simplified table comparing traditional lecture-based and active learning instructional processes

Aspect	Traditional lecture-based method	Active learning method
Teaching approach	Professor delivers a lecture; students passively listen	Students engage in discussions, problem-solving, and activities
Student role	Passive recipients of information	Active participants identifying learning needs and seeking answers
Assessment method	Focused on memorization and written exams	Includes presentations, peer discussions, and feedback
Knowledge retention	Often short-term and superficial	Deeper understanding with better long-term retention
Skill development	Limited to theoretical knowledge	Develops critical thinking, problem-solving, and application skills
Application of knowledge	Minimal opportunities for real-life application	Encourages practical use in realistic scenarios

5.4 Student Engagement as Active Members of the Institution

Just as there is benefit from students being active learners, there is benefit from students having an active role in institutional processes, decision-making, and planning. This role begins with an institutional culture that empowers students (Peters et al. 2019). Such a culture requires that there are policies and processes that support student involvement and includes individuals at all levels of an institution, including administrators and faculty, who are comfortable and supportive of student engagement. Students' involvement at the institutional level has benefits for students in terms of their development of leadership and other skills and for institutions in terms of contributions to quality improvement (Freitas et al. 2023). The following opportunities for student-institutional partnerships are considered important aspects of student engagement (Barzansky and Fuentealba 2024).

5.4.1 Engagement in Institutional Policy Development and Decision-Making

According to Schröder et al. (2020), active involvement in policy-making can result in better and more suitable educational policies if learners' opinions and experiences are considered and incorporated. Institutions can support student engagement in policy- and decision-making by having formal and codified roles for students to ensure that they are included in institutional committees and by providing mechanisms for students to respond to policies that affect educational programs and student life (Barzansky and Fuentealba 2024). It is helpful if institutional bylaws or other formal institutional documents specify which committees should include students.

The formal presence of students on committees ensures that the student voice will be present when issues relevant to the student body are considered. That voice is more credible if it reflects the opinions of the student body as a whole. It is, therefore, important to have mechanisms to collect input from the student body, both to inform student representatives to committees and to provide the opinion of students when it is requested by the administration on issues related to a proposed policy change. A formal student organization, such as a student council, can act as a conduit for information to and from the student body. Such a student organization can facilitate the collection of input from the entire study body. For example, the student council or class leaders can poll the student body to obtain student opinions quickly and comprehensively.

5.4.2 Engagement in Evaluation of Educational Programs

Students should be actively engaged in evaluating the curriculum. A comprehensive course evaluation system with a high student response rate ensures that student input is broad-based and representative. When responding to such evaluations, faculty action will be evidence-based and encourage students to continue to participate in providing evaluation data, as they see that their input leads to concrete and meaningful changes. In addition to evaluating general course content and instructional methods, students should evaluate individual teachers. Such evaluations are an important source of information for those responsible for the curriculum to ensure that faculty are creating an appropriate learning environment and are teaching with school and course expectations in mind. This information could also be used in faculty promotion and retention decisions, which would demonstrate active student engagement in ensuring educational program quality.

Students also need to be engaged in planning curriculum changes. As the group closest to the curriculum, student input can be valuable in identifying beneficial changes to curriculum and course organization and delivery (Peters et al. 2019). Techniques to collect student input could include surveys, class/student body meetings, and the inclusion of students on the planning committee.

5.4.3 Engagement in the Academic Environment

There are numerous roles that students can take to be engaged in the academic environment. These can support positive outcomes for the students themselves and for those with whom they engage.

Active learning involves students taking responsibility for their own learning. Students can also support the learning of their peers, for example, as tutors, coaches, or developers of instructional materials that are shared with their classmates. Peer teaching has been recommended as an institutional requirement, as it has positive results for both the students who provide instruction and those who receive it (Peters et al. 2019). Institutional support is important when students are preparing to be tutors and coaches. For example, faculty can orient students to the tutoring process and can ensure that their knowledge is sufficient and up-to-date. Faculty or student support staff can help orient students towards being effective coaches or mentors.

Participation in research and other scholarly activities is another way that students can be actively engaged in the academic environment. This engagement can take two primary forms: collaboration with faculty in support of their research and independent student-initiated research (Lombardi et al. 2021). Faculty collaboration involves interaction with individuals who have existing research programs, enabling students to learn first-hand how experts in a given field undertake research. Students gain practical knowledge from their mentors about research methodology and research skills, such as writing research papers. In this case, students would need institutional assistance in identifying a faculty mentor, and the mentor may need financial or other support for student participation. For self-generated research topics, students develop a research question, design a research plan to answer the question, gather data, and develop a conclusion. In addition to improving their familiarity with the material, they acquire various important skills, including problem-solving, critical thinking, and data analysis skills (Lombardi et al. 2021). Student-generated research requires institutional resources, such as space and funding, in addition to education in research design and data analysis to prepare them for their project. Both collaborative and self-generated research constitute other examples of active learning. Schools may require student research as part of the curriculum. In both required and voluntary research, the school can provide time for students to engage in research, such as during the summer when the school is not in session or during times set aside for electives. Schools can also provide support for students to present their research at meetings.

5.4.4 Engagement in the Community

Students may engage with the community in a variety of ways that both support their own learning and professional development and provide benefits to their community partners. Service learning/community service can be an institutional requirement or an elective volunteer opportunity. Typically, developing a community service experience involves gaining an understanding of community needs and creating activities to address them. The services delivered by health profession students should be appropriate for their educational and experience levels. Depending on the educational program, services may be health related, such as providing education to children about the dangers of smoking or staffing a free clinic under faculty supervision. Service may also involve raising funding to meet a specific community need. In any case, these activities allow students to gain leadership and team-building skills by developing and implementing the support program with their peers. Such involvement helps them understand the health-related and social context of the local environment (Jones et al. 2019).

5.5 Overcoming Barriers to Student Engagement

Barriers to student engagement, including active learning, fall into two general categories: institutional culture and logistical and implementation issues.

5.5.1 Institutional Culture

A collaborative organizational culture that is grounded in supportive institutional values is central to student engagement (Freitas et al. 2023). If faculty and administrators value students as partners, student engagement can be enhanced. Creating such a culture requires that the benefits to both faculty and students are apparent through, for example, communication channels that link students to their peers and students to faculty (Peters et al. 2019). Overcoming resistance is more likely in an environment where there is evidence of positive outcomes from student engagement. One such example would be curriculum changes based on student input that result in higher student satisfaction and enhanced student performance or evidence that a collaborative culture makes the school more attractive to applicants.

5.5.2 Logistical and Implementation Issues

There can be logistical challenges to incorporating student engagement into the learning environment. For example, student engagement though active learning requires the availability of active learning classrooms that permit easy student-to-student interaction (Odum et al. 2021). The lack of small group rooms or large group rooms that can be configured to support students working with their peers can limit the incorporation of some active learning instructional formats. For active learning to be successful, faculty need to be trained in those methods and be knowledgeable about different active learning formats. For example, an insufficient number of trained faculty facilitators for small group sessions and for providing students with feedback could be a barrier. Institutional commitment to student engagement may help alleviate these barriers through funding for facility renovations, if needed, or through identifying small group teaching spaces on campuses. The identification of additional faculty or increased time provided by existing faculty could also benefit from institutional funding.

Finding the time for students to engage as committee members, peer tutors and mentors, and researchers can be a barrier if the demands of the formal curriculum are heavy. Additionally, some active learning formats, such as problem-based learning and team-based learning, require students to work outside formal class time, such as looking up information to answer their questions or completing learning modules that will be discussed in class. Given these potential barriers, faculty need to set guidelines regarding the amount of time that will be available during the week, and students should have the opportunity to provide information on their workload to ensure that the guidelines are followed.

5.6 Conclusion

Student engagement should be an integral component of the learning environment in health professions. Ensuring this engagement requires a commitment from both schools and students. For educational institutions, that commitment comes through an organizational environment that provides opportunities for students to be engaged at multiple levels and the resources to support that engagement. Students must be willing to devote time to engagement activities. Together, these efforts can result in the reciprocal belief that the resources and time for student engagement are well spent in relation to students' professional development and their future roles as healthcare providers.

5.7 Short Chapter Summary

This chapter delves into the concept of student engagement in health profession education, emphasizing its significance in fostering lifelong learning and professional development. It highlights two key dimensions of engagement: active learning, where students take responsibility for their education, and active participation in institutional processes. Active learning is defined as a method where students are not passive recipients but active participants in their learning journey, using techniques such as problem-solving, discussions, and practical assignments to enhance comprehension and retention. Examples of active learning in medical education, like the transition from traditional lectures to case-based discussions, demonstrate its effectiveness in improving outcomes.

This chapter also underscores the value of student-institution partnerships, advocating for students' roles in institutional policy-making, curriculum evaluation, research, and community service. These partnerships are shown to benefit both students, by developing leadership and critical thinking skills, and institutions, by fostering quality improvement and innovation.

Barriers to engagement, such as institutional culture and logistical challenges, are analysed. Recommendations include fostering a collaborative culture, providing adequate resources, and training faculty and students to support engagement activities.

Ultimately, this chapter argues that student engagement should be a foundational element of the learning environment in health professions. Through mutual commitment from institutions and students, engagement can lead to enhanced educational quality, better professional preparedness, and a robust foundation for addressing the dynamic challenges of healthcare practice. This comprehensive approach ensures that students not only excel academically but are also well-equipped to contribute meaningfully to their fields.

References

Barzansky B, Fuentealba C. ASPIRE for excellence in student engagement: examples of how institutions operationalize a complex construct. Med Teach. 2024;47:617–21. https://doi.org/10.1080/0142159x.2024.2368565.

Freitas F, Leedham-Green KE, Smith SF, Costa MJ. Partners in academic endeavour: characterising student engagement across internationally excellent medical schools. Med Teach. 2023;45:830–7.

Gavarkovs AG, Finan E, Jensen RD, Brydges R. When I say … active learning. Med Educ. 2024;58:896–7.

Gareth J. Jones, Michael B. Edwards, Jason N. Bocarro, Per G. Svensson, Katie Misener. A community capacity building approach to sport-based youth development. Sport Management Review. 2019;23. https://doi.org/10.1016/j.smr.2019.09.001.

Kassab SE, Taylor D, Hamdy H. Student engagement in health professions education: AMEE guide no. 152. Med Teach. 2023;45:949–65.

Lombardi D, Shipley TF, Bailey JM, Bretones PS, Prather EE, Ballen CJ, Knight JK, Smith MK, Stowe RL, Cooper MM, Prince M, Atit K, Uttal DH, LaDue ND, McNeal PM, Ryker K, St. John K, Van Der Hoeven Kraft KJ, Docktor JL. The curious construct of active learning. Psychol Sci Public Interest. 2021;22:8–43.

Michael J. Where's the evidence that active learning works? Adv Physiol Educ. 2006;30:159–67.

Odum M, Meaney KS, Knudson DV. Active learning classroom design and student engagement: an exploratory study. J Learn Spaces. 2021;10:27–41.

Peters H, Zdravkovic M, Costa MJ, Celenza A, Ghias K, Klamen D, Mossop L, Rieder M, Nadarajah VD, Wangsaturaka D, Wohlin M, Weggemans M. Twelve tips for enhancing student engagement. Med Teach. 2019;41:632–7.

Schröder LMU, Wals AEJ, Van Koppen CSA. Analysing the state of student participation in two eco-schools using Engeström's second generation activity systems model. Environ Educ Res. 2020;26:1088–111.

The Art of Problem-Based Learning in the Context of Education in the Health Professions

6

Khalid A. Bin Abdulrahman, Lulu Abdulrahman Alwazzan, and Hassan Darami

Learning Objectives

1. Understand the principles of problem-based learning (PBL).
   - Learners will be able to identify and explain the key principles of PBL, including authenticity, active learning, patient-centeredness, and differentiation, and how these principles enhance healthcare education.
2. Apply techniques associated with PBL.
   - Learners will demonstrate the ability to utilize PBL techniques, such as student-centered learning, integrating basic and clinical sciences, problem-solving, critical thinking, and reflection, to address complex healthcare scenarios.
3. Analyze the benefits and challenges of PBL implementation.
   - Learners will critically evaluate the advantages of PBL in fostering critical thinking, collaboration, and self-directed learning, as well as identify and address potential challenges in its implementation within healthcare education.

K. A. Bin Abdulrahman (✉) · L. A. Alwazzan
Department of Medical Education, College of Medicine, Imam Mohammad Ibn Saud Islamic University (IMSIU), Riyadh, Saudi Arabia
e-mail: kab@imamu.edu.sa; laalwazzan@imamu.edu.sa

H. Darami
Department of Obstetrics & Gynecology and Medical Education, College of Medicine, Imam Mohammad Ibn Saud Islamic University (IMSIU), Riyadh, Saudi Arabia
e-mail: hwdarami@imamu.edu.sa

K. A. Bin Abdulrahman, H. Darami (eds.), *Essential Learning Skills for Health Professions Students*, https://doi.org/10.1007/978-981-96-5670-7_6

6.1 Introduction

Learning has always been a critical component of healthcare as a result of its impacts on the nature and quality of services offered throughout this industry. Healthcare professionals are required to optimize their knowledge, skills, and attitudes with the goal of ensuring the best possible outcomes for their patients. As such, relevant actors in this profession must be aware of key learning needs in this context. While conventional teacher-led learning continues to dominate the profession, insights into the impacts of this approach have revealed that it must be updated to address emerging needs in healthcare.

One of the most accessible learning techniques that can replace teacher-led learning is problem-based learning (PBL). PBL is a cornerstone of modern education in the health professions, which has revolutionized traditional pedagogical approaches by placing learners at the center of their educational journey. The value of PBL lies in its emphasis on problem-solving and critical thinking skills that remain essential in the context of education in the health professions. PBL immerses students in authentic, real-world scenarios that enable them to cope with complex health issues, to simulate clinical encounters, and to collaborate to develop solutions.

6.2 Principles and Techniques Associated with PBL

6.2.1 Principles

Problem-based learning is characterized by various principles that highlight its superior ability to equip healthcare professionals with novel forms of knowledge and skills. The first principle associated with PBL is authenticity. PBL focuses on imparting knowledge and skills that are relevant to the real world (Henderson 2016). Proponents of this learning model have claimed that learners can acquire more knowledge and insights into their practice if they are informed of the problems that they can encounter throughout their clinical practice. The second principle associated with PBL is an emphasis on active learning. Conventional learning mechanisms encourage learners to be mere recipients of knowledge and skills; however, this approach has proven to be inadequate in light of the different needs and capabilities of learners (Merrou et al. 2023). Hence, new strategies must be adopted to enable learners to explore their abilities during the learning process. PBL shifts the focus of this process from the passive reception of information to active engagement with content. Students serve as self-directed learners, explore topics, conduct searches, and collaborate with their peers to solve problems.

Patient-centeredness and differentiation represent the other principles associated with PBL. Healthcare professionals learn and acquire novel skills and knowledge with the aim of ensuring the best possible outcomes for their patients. As such, the principle of patient-centeredness is in line with the primary mandate of education in the health professions

(Merrou et al. 2023). Accordingly, PBL places patients at the center of the learning experience, thereby emphasizing the importance of patient care, empathy, and professionalism in this context. By engaging with authentic patient cases, students develop a deeper understanding of the human dimensions of healthcare and cultivate patient-centered attitudes and behaviors. Finally, PBL is associated with the principle of differentiation. Conventionally, educators treat all learners equally. Conventional learning techniques thus emphasize a collective approach to knowledge acquisition. This emphasis has changed in the context of PBL, which encourages teachers to recognize that students learn at different paces and exhibit different strengths and weaknesses. As such, teachers must tailor instructions to meet the individual needs of each student. In line with these principles, PBL represents a more coherent and relevant approach to contemporary needs in healthcare settings.

6.2.2 Techniques

A variety of techniques have been incorporated into PBL with the aim of addressing emerging learning needs in contemporary healthcare settings. The most notable of such technique is student-centered learning. This technique, which is also known as learner-centered education, is an instructional approach that shifts the focus of this process from the teacher to the student. In a traditional classroom, the teacher is the primary source of information, including by delivering lectures and assigning exercises (Badge et al. 2024). In a student-centered classroom, students play a more active role in the learning process. Student-centered learning involves several key techniques, including student choice, according to which students have more control over what they learn and how they learn it. Such control could involve choosing topics to explore, selecting projects to complete, or making decisions concerning learning activities. Student-centered learning also encompasses student responsibility, which encourages learners to take ownership of their learning by setting goals, tracking their progress, and reflecting on their achievements. Student-centered learning is also characterized by active learning that allows students to engage in activities that promote critical thinking, problem-solving, and collaboration. This approach might involve project-based learning, discussions, simulations, or games. Ultimately, this technique entails differentiation, such that the unique needs of all students are accommodated on the basis of their strengths and weaknesses.

The second technique that characterizes PBL pertains to the integration of skills in both basic and clinical sciences. PBL aims to bridge the gap between basic scientific knowledge and clinical application. The objective of this learning method is to equip learners with the best understanding of clinical settings (García-Sierra et al. 2024). As such, by contextualizing theoretical concepts with regard to clinical scenarios, PBL enhances learners' ability to understand and retain foundational knowledge while reinforcing the relevance of such knowledge to clinical practice. To ensure that the learners acquire the required skills, PBL involves continuous assessments and feedback (Badge et al. 2024). Assessments in the context of PBL are ongoing and multifaceted, and they pertain to both individual and group performance. Regular feedback from facilitators and peers allows students to monitor their progress, identify areas of strength and weakness, and refine their problem-solving strategies.

Additional techniques have been absorbed into PBL in light of its objective of addressing the unique needs of learners. One such technique involves emphasizing problem-solving and critical thinking skills (García-Sierra et al. 2024). PBL is a learning technique that seeks to cultivate both hands-on and theoretical knowledge acquisition. This multifaceted approach is rooted in the inputs provided by learners in their efforts to solve various problems while using critical thinking to identify appropriate solutions. Hence, students analyze complex clinical cases, identify relevant information, generate hypotheses, and evaluate evidence with the goals of producing diagnoses and proposing treatment plans. Similarly, students are engaged in a process of inquiry-based learning (Badge et al. 2024). That is, PBL learning involves asking students questions, seeking answers, and engaging in self-directed exploration of topics. This approach fosters curiosity, self-motivation, and a lifelong commitment to learning. Finally, the technique emphasizes reflection. Reflection is integral to the PBL process, thereby allowing students to assess their learning, identify areas for improvement, and integrate new knowledge with prior experiences (Narong and Hallinger 2023). Additionally, through reflection, students develop metacognitive awareness and enhance their ability to adapt to evolving challenges in the field of healthcare. Other auxiliary techniques that have been implemented in the context of PBL include facilitator guidance and interdisciplinary collaboration, which combine to allow learners to master a wider scope with regard to their practice.

6.3 The PBL Process

The PBL process refers to the key steps involved in the process of engaging learners through the implementation of various techniques pertaining to PBL. To streamline this process, consider a common clinical scenario featuring Mr. Ali, a high school teacher, who is experiencing unexpected chest pain (see Fig. 6.1).

The first step in the process involves identifying the problem. This step should pertain to a well-defined scenario or case study (Narong and Hallinger 2023). This scenario should, in turn, reflect a real-world situation that health professionals might encounter. The facilitator encourages the students to examine the scenario critically. The learning objective at this stage is to allow students to identify key details, relevant medical history, and potential areas of concern pertaining to the case. This initial analysis helps students grasp the core issue and prepare for further investigation. The problem identification stage offers a range of benefits, including increased engagement in the learning process. That is, a captivating case should capture students' attention and motivate them to engage more deeply with the topic at hand. This step also allows the knowledge gaps among learners to

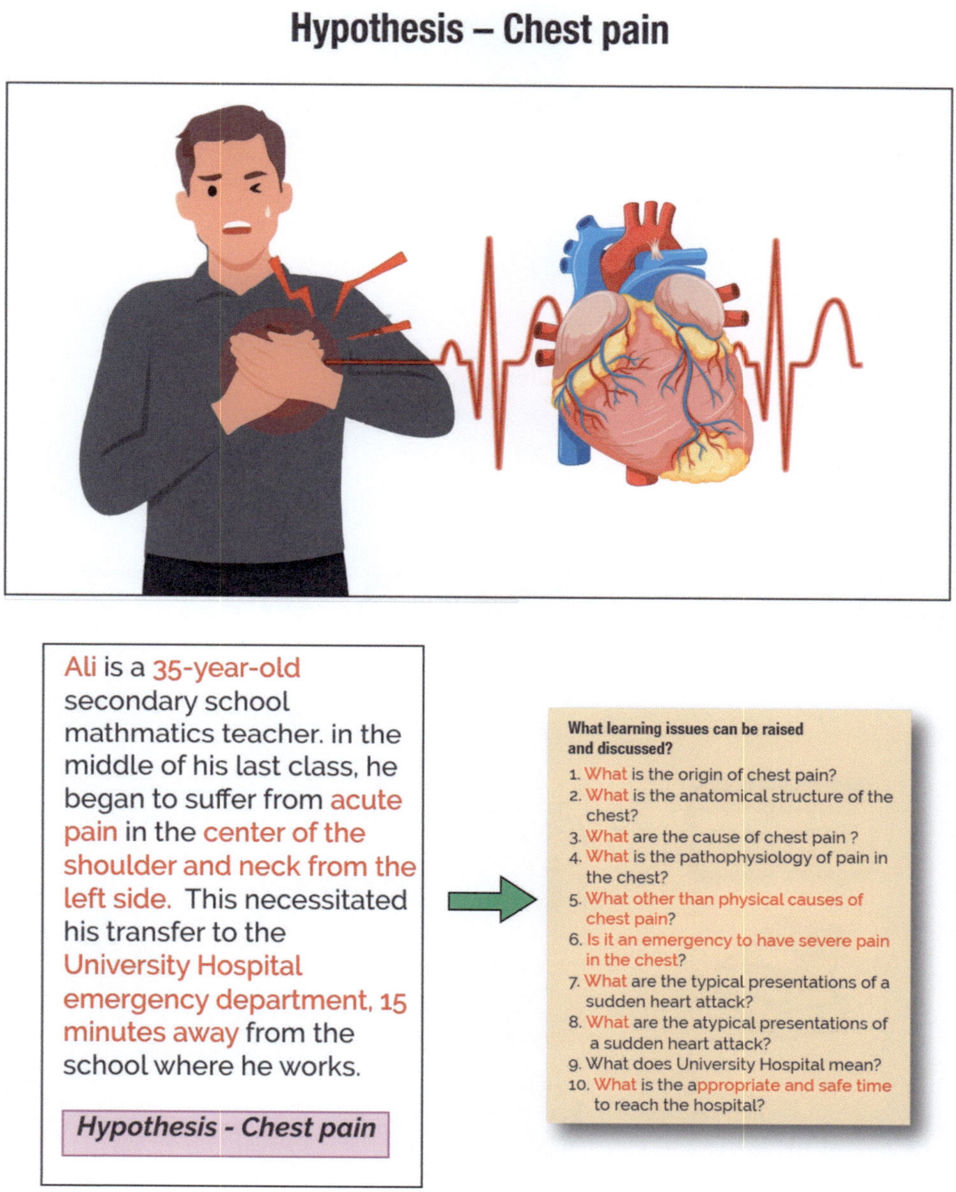

Fig. 6.1 An example of PBL case scenario

be identified. Namely, this step allows learners to assess the problem, thereby allowing them to recognize aspects that require further exploration. Figure 6.2 illustrates the process of PBL tutorial.

The second step in PBL involves analyzing the problem. During this stage, learners are allowed to work collaboratively to explore and deconstruct the problem at hand.

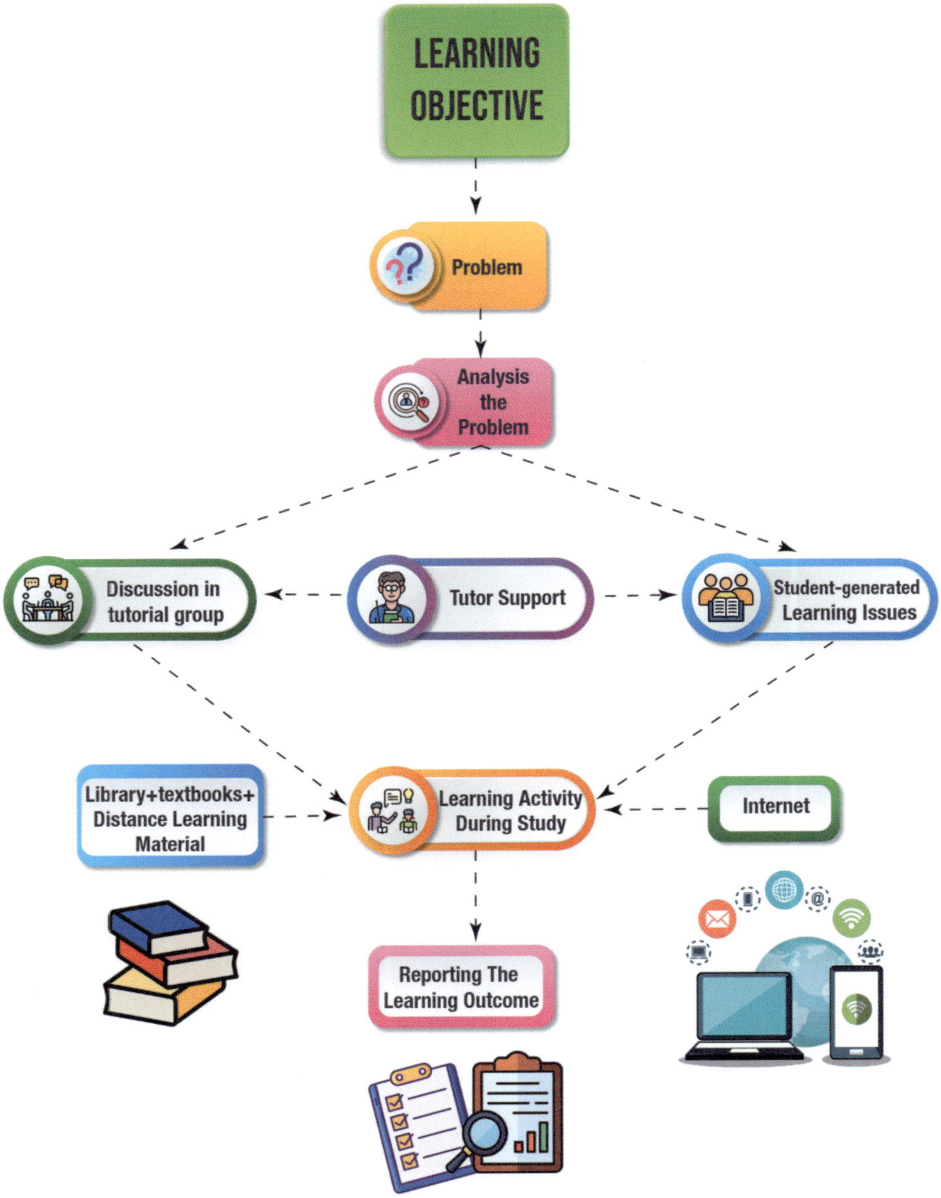
LEARNING OBJECTIVE
Problem
Analysis the Problem
Discussion in tutorial group
Tutor Support
Student-generated Learning Issues
Library+textbooks+ Distance Learning Material
Learning Activity During Study
Internet
Reporting The Learning Outcome

Fig. 6.2 An illustration of the process of PBL tutorial

The objective of this stage is to outline the varying approaches that learners employ in their attempts to understand or address the problem (Narong and Hallinger 2023). As such, students engage in brainstorming regarding potential causes, identify relevant factors, and consider different perspectives during this stage with the goal of

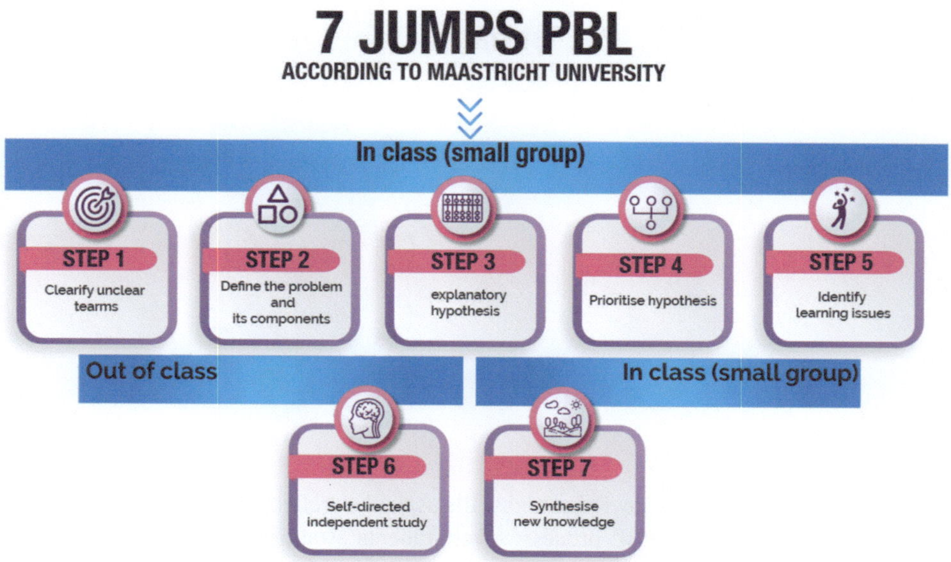

Fig. 6.3 The seven-jump model of the PBL process

addressing the problem. Notably, this stage encourages critical thinking, communication, and collaboration, as students work together to gain a deeper understanding of the issue at hand. This stage is important for two reasons. First, it helps learners develop critical thinking skills. Namely, it allows learners to participate in key activities that include analyzing information, identifying key aspects, and considering various viewpoints. Second, this stage fosters collaboration. In this context, learners are allowed to work together, thereby strengthening their communication and teamwork skills. Figure 6.3 demonstrates the Maastricht seven-jump model of the PBL process (Wood 2003; Albanese and Mitchell 2010).

The third step in this process involves formulating a learning plan. In light of previously identified deficiencies in understanding and knowledge gaps, learners are allowed to construct a study strategy during this stage (Nagel et al. 2024). This strategy highlights the precise knowledge and competencies that learners need to address this issue competently. Additionally, learners might identify specific references such as textbooks, scholarly papers, or digital repositories for consultation. This methodical learning strategy guarantees a concentrated and effective method that can be used to acquire expertise. This third step is vital for two reasons. Primarily, allowing learners to formulate individualistic plans encourages them to engage in self-directed learning and develop their information literacy skills. Second, an emphasis on this step helps promote learners' effective time management and organizational skills (Fig. 6.4 illustrates the standard configuration of the interactions that occur among participants during a typical PBL session).

Fig. 6.4 Setup of PBL tutorial

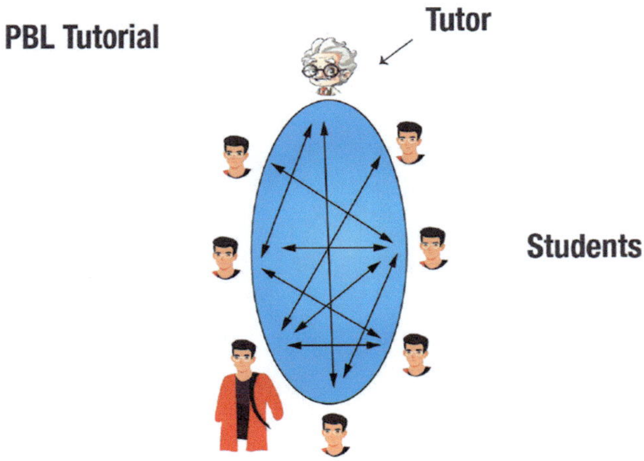

The acquisition of new knowledge and skills as well as reflection and evaluation represent the final stages of the PBL process. After students establish a well-defined learning plan, they proactively pursue the required knowledge and skills. This phase entails self-directed study, collaborative dialogues, and potential lectures delivered by healthcare experts. On this basis, students critically assess the information that they encounter and combine it with their preexisting knowledge to obtain a better understanding of the issue under investigation. This stage offers various benefits to learners, including enhanced knowledge retention through active learning and opportunities for collaboration and peer learning (Nagel et al. 2024). The final stage of this process involves reflection and evaluation, in which context students reconsider the initial problem in light of their newfound knowledge. They discuss potential solutions, evaluate the effectiveness of their learning plans, and identify areas for improvement. Such reflection allows students to consolidate their learning and develop their metacognitive skills, which refer to the ability to think about their thinking. This final stage is also important, as it reinforces key concepts and enables students to obtain a deeper understanding. Furthermore, it provides an opportunity to assess learning outcomes and identify areas for further development. Every participant in a PBL academic session must have mastered and continue to adhere to their assigned role. Figure 6.5 summarizes the roles played by PBL participants during such a session (El Naggar et al. 2013).

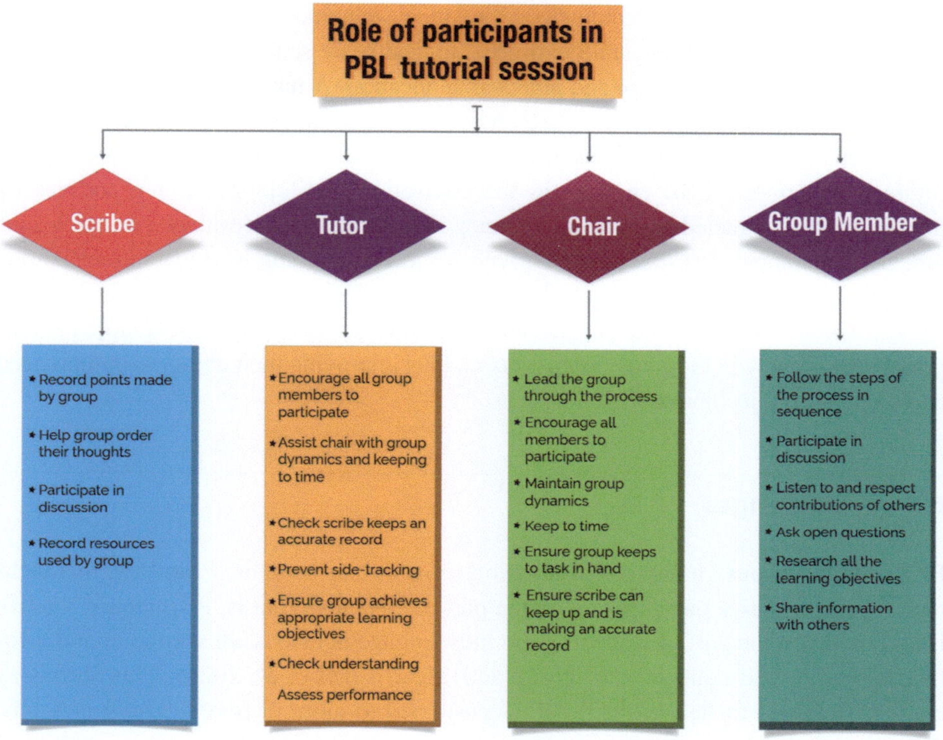

Fig. 6.5 Roles of all participants in PBL tutorial. (Source: El Naggar et al. 2013)

6.4 Benefits and Challenges of PBL

6.4.1 Benefits

The implementation of PBL in a professional learning setting offers a range of benefits. Most notably, this method enhances critical thinking and problem-solving skills among learners (Nagel et al. 2024). That is, through PBL, students become actively involved in the processes of dissecting authentic situations, performing critical analysis, identifying pivotal concerns, and formulating evidence-based solutions. This practice enhances their capacity to address intricate problems in a skillful manner. PBL also promotes augmented self-guided learning and cooperation. Namely, PBL allows students to take responsibility for their own educational journey, particularly by highlighted areas in which their knowledge is deficient and encouraging them to acquire information proactively (Amir et al. 2024). By extension, this technique emphasizes collaboration within teams with the goal of promoting effective communication, teamwork, and the capacity to draw insights from one's peers.

The practical application of knowledge and the development of lifelong skills are additional benefits of the implementation of PBL in healthcare settings. PBL bridges the gap between theoretical knowledge and practical application (Amir et al. 2024). As such, students acquire the ability to use their expertise to address authentic healthcare challenges, thus equipping them to address the professional contexts that they will encounter in the future. Furthermore, PBL emphasizes the cultivation of lifelong learning abilities by focusing on self-directed learning, proficiency in information retrieval, and research aptitude. These competencies are essential with respect to ongoing learning and adaptation throughout a career in the health professions. Finally, PBL often leads to higher levels of engagement and motivation than conventional lecture-based approaches. Hence, students participate actively in the educational process, thus improving their ability to comprehend and retain the subject matter.

6.5 Challenges

PBL entails various challenges in addition to its strong benefits. Primarily, this technique requires active participation on the part of students. That is, PBL requires active involvement on the part of students, who must engage in discussions, conduct independent research, and contribute to group activities (Nagel et al. 2024). This shift may entail difficulties for learners who are accustomed to more passive learning methods. Second, stakeholders must consider the extensive time investment requirements associated with the implementation of PBL. A comprehensive understanding of complex problems requires significant time investments. Hence, students may find it necessary to allocate extra time beyond the hours they spend in class to research, group collaboration, and reflection.

Additionally, this technique has the potential to lead to confusion and learner frustration. Namely, encountering unfamiliar scenarios or complex medical concepts may result in confusion or frustration among students (Amir et al. 2024). As such, effective facilitation and clearly defined learning objectives provide essential guidance for students in response to such challenges. Finally, the implementation of PBL may require an understanding of group dynamics. Collaborative work can entail various challenges. Students must cultivate effective communication and teamwork skills to establish a constructive group learning environment. Overall, PBL offers a valuable approach to education, but it is important to acknowledge the potential challenges that it entails. By providing students with proper support and guidance, educators can help them overcome these challenges and take advantage of the many benefits offered by PBL.

6.6 Effective PBL Implementation

Every attempt to implement PBL effectively entails various considerations. The first such consideration focuses on the evolution of team dynamics and the need to understand this process. The success of PBL depends strongly on how teams operate and how they achieve goals such as collective objectives (Walker et al. 2015). To promote effective team dynamics, learners and their facilitators must emphasize a range of factors. The first such factor is effective communication. It is important for every stakeholder in PBL to express their ideas clearly, listen actively to others, and remain open to different perspectives. The second factor pertaining to effective team dynamics is shared responsibility. Stakeholders must distribute tasks equally, hold each other accountable, and celebrate successes with one another (Nagel et al. 2024). Such activities can enhance the bonds among participants in a team. Additionally, respectful collaboration within teams is necessary. That is, team members must be encouraged to value diverse ideas, manage conflicts constructively, and focus on achieving a common goal. Ensuring that teams operate optimally is similar to the task of achieving the basic objectives of PBL.

The second consideration pertaining to the implementation of PBL focuses on the role of the facilitator. The facilitator plays a crucial role in guiding the PBL process. However, learning in this context ultimately remains student driven (Amir et al. 2024). Nevertheless, the facilitator can provide context and set expectations. Accordingly, the facilitator introduces the case study, outlines learning objectives, and establishes clear guidelines for group work. Second, the facilitator should guide discussions and inquiries. The facilitator should also ask thought-provoking questions to encourage critical thinking and steer the conversation toward a deeper understanding. Moreover, the facilitator should steer the process of resource acquisition. He or she can help identify relevant resources such as textbooks, online databases, or guest speakers. Finally, the facilitator's role involves providing support and feedback. The facilitator offers guidance throughout the process, answers questions, and helps students stay on track. Additionally, the facilitator assesses the students with the goal of obtaining a deeper understanding of their capabilities.

During the process of implementing PBL, stakeholders should consider the development of effective learning plans. A well-structured learning plan ensures that students can acquire the necessary knowledge and skills. Such plans can be developed on the basis of an initial identification of relevant knowledge gaps. On the basis of a case study analysis, stakeholders can identify the specific topics or concepts about which they must learn more. The second strategy should involve setting smart, measurable, attainable, relevant, and time-bound (SMART) goals (Amir et al. 2024), which is important during the learning process. This approach helps anchor the process exclusively in purposes pertaining to learning. To set well-structured goals, learners must only adhere to the objectives of PBL throughout the process.

Additionally, learners must choose appropriate resources during the process of implementing PBL. The field of healthcare is vast, and the task of navigating the abundance of information that characterizes this field can be overwhelming (Henderson 2016). To choose appropriate resources, learners can thus utilize textbooks, research articles, and online databases or consult with the facilitator to obtain guidance concerning relevant resources. Scheduling time for learning and tracking progress are additional strategies that should be considered in the context of efforts to implement PBL. Learners must allocate dedicated time for research, group discussions, and individual studies on the basis of their goals and the relevant project timeline (Merrou et al. 2023). Finally, learners should monitor their learning journey by taking notes, summarizing key concepts, and identifying areas that require further exploration.

6.7 Final Thoughts and Summary

Learning in each industry is a changing process. For example, healthcare focuses on developing learning techniques that can address both current and future needs. Notably, PBL is a unique learning method that can revitalize the processes of knowledge acquisition and dissemination in healthcare. Namely, PBL emphasizes the needs of the learners and exposes those learners to real-world applications. Additionally, PBL is relatively flexible, thus allowing it to accommodate a range of learning techniques. Importantly, consideration of different stakeholder roles is necessary to ensure the efficient implementation of PBL. Notably, despite its multiple benefits, PBL also entails various challenges that must be addressed if its application is to be effective. Box 6.1 summarizes the final thoughts of the art of PBL.

Box 6.1 Final Thoughts

- Problem-based learning (PBL) is an innovative educational approach that has the potential to rejuvenate the process by which knowledge is acquired and shared in the field of healthcare.
- PBL prioritizes learners' requirements and exposes them to real-world applications.
- PBL can be easily adapted to a variety of learning methodologies.
- It is crucial to account for the various roles played by stakeholders in this context ensure the effective implementation of PBL.
- Importantly, despite its numerous advantages, PBL also entails various problems that must be resolved for its successful implementation.

References

Albanese MA, Mitchell S. Problem-based learning: a review of literature on its outcomes and implementation issues. Acad Med. 2010;85(5):778–84. https://doi.org/10.1097/ACM.0b013e3181d5ef14.

Amir M, Hassan N, Khalid U. Enhancing medical education: a pathway to nurturing future healthcare professionals. Cureus. 2024;16:e51920.

Badge A, Chandankhede M, Gajbe U, Bankar NJ, Bandre GR. Employment of small-group discussions to ensure the effective delivery of medical education. Cureus. 2024;16:e52655.

García-Sierra R, Fernández-Cano MI, Jiménez-Pera M, Feijoo-Cid M, Marañón AA. Knowledge about the best practice guidelines in the nursing degree: a non-randomized post-test design. Nurs Open. 2024;11:e2074.

Henderson R. Problem-based learning: perspectives methods and challenges. New York: Nova Science Publisher's; 2016.

Merrou S, Jouicha AI, Baslam A, Ouhaz Z, El Adib AR. Problem-based learning method in the context of a flipped classroom: outcomes on pain management course acquisition. Asia Pac Sch. 2023;8:5–12.

Nagel DA, Penner JL, Halas G, Philip MT, Cooke CA. Exploring experiential learning within interprofessional practice education initiatives for pre-licensure healthcare students: a scoping review. BMC Med Educ. 2024;24:139.

Naggar E, Abd MA, Aziz E. Effectiveness of implementing a tutor training workshop for problem based learning class tutors at the faculty of medicine, Suez Canal University. Intellect Prop Rights. 2013;1:1000104.

Narong DK, Hallinger P. A keyword co-occurrence analysis of research on service learning: conceptual foci and emerging research trends. Educ Sci. 2023;13:339.

Walker A, Leary H, Hmelo-Silver C, Ertmer P. Essential readings in problem-based learning. USA: Purdue University Press; 2015.

Wood DF. ABC of learning and teaching in medicine: problem-based learning. BMJ. 2003;326(7384):328–30. https://doi.org/10.1136/bmj.326.7384.328.

How to Be an Effective, Self-Directed Learner

7

Khalid A. Bin Abdulrahman

Learning Objectives

1. *Understand the core principles of self-directed learning (SDL).*
   Learners will be able to define SDL, identify its key components, and explain its significance in fostering autonomy, motivation, and lifelong learning skills.
2. *Develop and apply SDL strategies.*
   Learners will learn how to set SMART objectives, create effective study plans, utilize diverse resources, and engage in self-assessment and reflection to enhance their educational and professional growth.
3. *Overcome challenges and adapt SDL to varied contexts.*
   Learners will be equipped to address common SDL challenges, such as isolation and lack of discipline, and adapt SDL principles to different learning environments and career development scenarios.

7.1 Introduction

Self-directed learning (SDL) represents the most significant shift in educational paradigms; in this context, the learner plays a core developmental role. This revolutionary approach reforms the identity of the conventional education system, according to which educators enrol, train, and manage learners. Unlike traditional approaches to learning, which are more rigid and require little more than receptiveness, *SDL* is participatory and individualized, thereby requiring the student to take ownership of the learning process. When learners are accountable for decisions regarding learning, such as the selection of

K. A. Bin Abdulrahman (✉)
Department of Medical Education, College of Medicine, Imam Mohammad Ibn Saud Islamic University (IMSIU), Riyadh, Saudi Arabia
e-mail: kab@imamu.edu.sa

K. A. Bin Abdulrahman, H. Darami (eds.), *Essential Learning Skills for Health Professions Students*, https://doi.org/10.1007/978-981-96-5670-7_7

the content, rate, and approach included in the learning process, they are more likely to be committed; accordingly, they can obtain a richer and more effective education. *SDL* is characterized by the transformation of conventional educators into mentors and tutors, who engage learners as discoverers rather than as followers (Loeng 2020). Not only does this independence encourage learners to exhibit more significant effort; these individuals also become more personally invested in the learning content. Therefore, such content may be more relevant to their world. Accordingly, in addition to its direct educational effects, *SDL* fosters vital life skills, including problem-solving, critical thinking, and self-education skills, throughout learners' lifetime. These skills become more essential as knowledge becomes more dynamic and when some of the competencies that are essential in the workplace are instilled in members of the millennial generation (Vincent-Lancrin 2023).

In this chapter, we discuss pragmatic approaches to *SDL* as well as the numerous benefits of this approach, and we provide learners who are willing to improve their *SDL* abilities with a clear, step-by-step guide to this process. This chapter expands on the ways in which learners can initiate and maintain *SDL* engagement by establishing goals and objectives, recognizing appropriate sources, and becoming organized while following a plan. The narrative includes the steps that should be taken in the process of searching actively for feedback as well as the significance of self-evaluation regarding whether the learner is on the right track or whether the learner should modify the strategies that he or she uses. This emphasis on practical application and case studies reveals how *SDL* can positively affect various areas at different phases of individuals' lives. It also highlights issues that self-directed learners may face, such as isolation and a lack of discipline, as well as possible solutions to these problems.

7.2 Defining SDL and Understanding Its Importance

SDL is a learning model in which a learner is responsible for identifying relevant learning needs or objectives as well as appropriate ways, means, and times to learn. This educational model focuses intensely on the individual learner, thus identifying the concept of choice as the primary determinant of the individual's educational path. This kind of autonomy is not simply an option that is equivalent to choice-making; rather, it is a tremendous responsibility that enables learners to become more personally involved, thus increasing their motivation and commitment. When learners can decide what and how they want to learn, they tend to be more responsible than in situations in which the teacher compels them to behave in a certain way. This sense of responsibility is essential because it helps learners develop attitudes that can be compounded by passion, thus making them likely to read and overcome any barriers they may encounter (Loeng 2020). Moreover, *SDL* enforces positive personal attitudes, which are helpful with respect to the need to attend classes and learn throughout one's life, including in different life situations. Given its role in the task of offering learners control over their learning experience, *SDL* encompasses the inherent benefits of a learner-controlled learning environment and a direction that is in line with the learner's educational plans as well as the learner's future goals (Morris et al. 2023).

The significance of autonomy in *SDL* lays a foundation for an elaborate concept of individualized learning, which is another advantage offered by this model of education. Thus, flexible learning can be described as the individual's ability to fine-tune his or her method of studying in a way that depends on his or her own learning style, aptitudes, and speed preferences. This approach thus represents a significant response to learners' heterogeneous needs, interests, goals, and variability in terms of cultural experiences (Loeng 2020). For example, specific learners may be comfortable with graphics, videos, and online tutorials, whereas others may prefer interactive groups or kinaesthetic projects. Thus, through such individualization, *SDL* increases the efficiency of educational activities and renders the learning process meaningful and comprehensible (Gilakjani 2012). Hence, it entails that learning becomes active rather than passive, thus enabling citizens to learn in a way to which they can relate both personally and professionally. Furthermore, this tailored approach lays a foundation for an additional crucial aspect of *SDL*: the adequate application of a variety of educational resources, which can expand the learning environment and facilitate students' general development (Loeng 2020; Morris et al. 2023).

7.2.1 Advantages of SDL

The opportunity and freedom associated with *SDL* extend far beyond flexibility in an academic setting; this approach can profoundly improve the individuals' development both as an individual and in his or her career. *SDL* influences motivation by allowing learners to choose the topics and objectives that are most meaningful to them. This *intrinsic motivation* is important because it allows learners to explore books in depth and seek more resources that they can use to respond to difficulties that emerge during the learning process. Since learning occurs when people are interested in a given topic for their own sakes, people invest more effort and resources into the process of becoming educated, thus making learning more satisfying and meaningful. Additionally, this motivation applies to educational environments and can easily be transferred into working life, as people are encouraged to act proactively and to become self-starters.

In addition to motivation, *SDL* helps improve the process of knowledge preservation. Learners who can take control of their learning procedures prefer techniques that are in line with their own learning styles, which entails that the techniques used in the learning process can enhance their ability to absorb and implement knowledge efficiently. When visuals, demonstrations, experiments, or discussions are used, *SDL* enables the learner to engage with information in a way that makes that content easy to understand and thus memorable. In addition to making learning fun, this approach provides a system through which individuals can retain the knowledge that they have acquired for longer, which is essential with regard to their continuing education and professional development. In addition, *SDL* equips learners with the flexibility they need to succeed in any learning setting. They become capable of adapting to learning situations on the basis of the environment and the available materials; this capability is thus highly desirable in the contemporary world. Such adaptability is necessary not only in educational or occupational environments but also in the process of becoming, in which context a person's ability to learn and change is crucial with regard to their efforts to improve their quality of life and manage intricate life circumstances. This seamless transition between different learning contexts highlights another significant aspect of *SDL*: the establishment of a *synergistic learning environment* that becomes possible when the right organizational learning tools and techniques are used appropriately.

7.3 Strategies for Becoming an Effective, Self-Directed Learner

7.3.1 Utilization of SMART Objectives

The first process involved in *SDL* is goal setting because this step provides direction and a way of measuring accomplishments. The goals in question must be clear and quantifiable in terms of the expected results associated with the plan; furthermore, they must be realistic and in line with the relevant business strategy, and the plan must include time-bound objectives. This method directs learners' focus to the material at hand and enhances their motivation because every completed segment elicits a feeling of accomplishment and thus facilitates more learning (Chatterjee and Corral 2017).

7.3.2 Developing a Study Plan

The structure of a typical study plan or timetable is presented in Table 7.1. In this context, the arrangement of the study period is necessary with respect to time organization and in light of the need to ensure that all the necessary study materials are covered sufficiently. This process entails developing the content that is to be taught, the time that is to be allocated to the learning process in light of the degree of difficulty and complexity associated with the relevant content, and the incorporation of predefined check-points to confirm that progress has been made (Yen et al. 2018). The ability to include variation in the general structure of studies to permit changes or entry into typically exciting areas of a given field of study if necessary is also important. For example, a student in a computer science class may find that he or she is interested in machine learning. However, this student must take other online courses or perform other projects within that field. In this manner, the learning process can capitalize on the motivation or curiosity exhibited by the learner. In addition, when determining particular types of work, it is most important to include breaks for review, thus ensuring that learners can fully understand easier concepts as the work proceeds before they encounter more difficult concepts. This goal can be accomplished

Table 7.1 A sample study plan for a nursing student

Time	Day 1	Day 2	Day 3	Day 4	Day 5
15:00–16:00 16:00–17:00	Study theoretical knowledge pertaining to anatomy	Study theoretical knowledge pertaining to pharmacology	Study theoretical knowledge pertaining to physical assessment	Practice charting skills	Practice physical evaluation skills
17:00–18:00	Rest	Rest	Rest	Rest	Rest
18:00–19:00	Dinner	Dinner	Dinner	Dinner	Dinner
20:00–21:00	Study theoretical knowledge pertaining to physiology	Study theoretical knowledge pertaining to nursing essentials	Study theoretical knowledge pertaining to advanced cardiac life support (ACLS)	Practice ACLS	Practice nursing skills pertaining to bedside manoeuvres

through weekend recalls, in which the content taught during the previous week is likely to be reviewed, or through group studies with other students, in which context different students can quiz one another on relevant areas (Larabi-Marie-Sainte et al. 2021; Yen et al. 2018).

7.3.3 Using Multiple Resources

Different types of learning can improve and broaden the amount of information provided concerning the subject at hand. Various resources, such as computers, libraries, and expert speeches, can help learners improve their understanding and inform them of additional perspectives. For example, a student of environmental science may use academic publications to obtain new information, rely on documentaries for practical purposes, and participate in expert-led online conferences concerning contemporary concerns and possibilities. This mode of learning and the consolidation of knowledge via texts, videos, and other media render the learning process enjoyable. This approach thus enables learners to explore a given subject in further depth and to ensure that the knowledge thus acquired is applicable to their specific contexts across various learner preferences.

7.3.4 Feedback and Guidance

Figure 7.1 reveals that *intermittent feedback* is important with respect to efforts to review learning intervention strategies and optimize the corresponding results, which can provide significant help to learners. For example, a nurse or doctor participates in daily case review sessions or clinical simulations. They discuss the treatment strategies or methods they use in the context of specific procedures with their colleagues and instructors (Bürgermeister

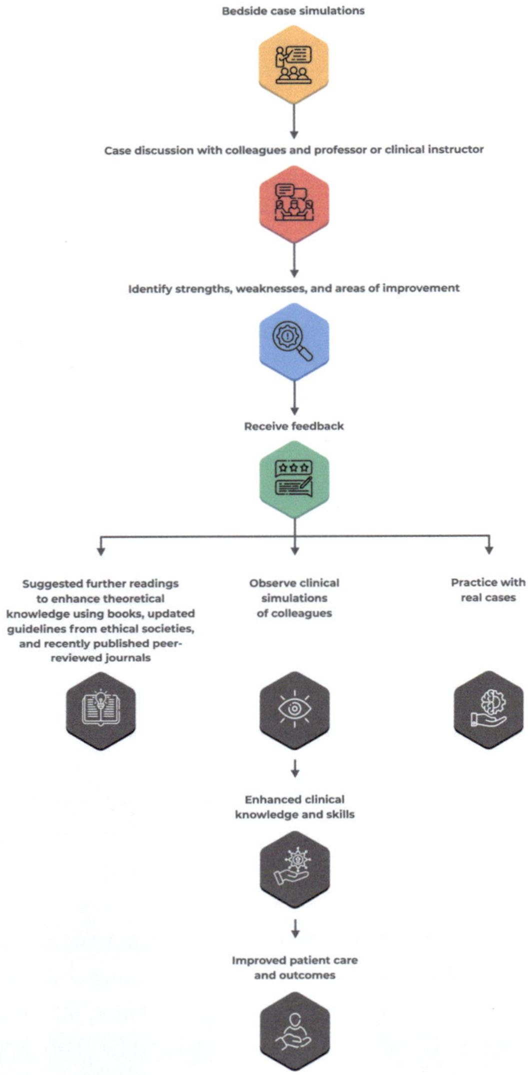

Fig. 7.1 Step-by-step process of providing feedback

et al. 2021). This approach enables them to become aware of their weaknesses with respect to clinical decision-making and practical clinical skills, thus allowing them to enhance patient care or procedural outcomes (Burgess et al. 2020). One aim of these sessions is to allow individuals to obtain essential feedback from mentors and colleagues, which can increase their clinical knowledge and guarantee that the learning process is in line with modern requirements (Henderson et al. 2019; Yang et al. 2021).

Furthermore, this approach is supported by the feedback provided alongside targeted instructions, which are crucial ways of helping medical professionals stay on a particular valuable and relevant track with regard to their further professional and continuing development. Such guidance may involve suggestions concerning other relevant texts, which contain further information regarding relevant cases, additional training, or participation in real cases that may be different from those that they have already encountered in the classroom (Henderson et al. 2019; Yang et al. 2021). These structured feedback mechanisms are essential in the medical field since constant education and development are critical with regard to efforts to address innovations in medical equipment and innovative aspects of particular treatment methods. By participating in these feedback loops, medical personnel can not only improve their skills and knowledge in terms of their working practices but also promote individual and organizational learning, thereby increasing their expertise and, consequently, improving patient care (Burgess et al. 2020; Nuuyoma 2021).

7.3.5 Self-Reflection and Self-Assessment

Figure 7.2 illustrates the fact that self-reflection and self-assessment are indispensable with regard to efforts to understand these processes and make any necessary modifications. The procedures associated with self-evaluation in the context of educators' and learners' experiences include reflective journal practice during the teaching and learning process, which can enable learners to understand their profound educational experiences. This practice refers to situations in which a student records his or her interactions with various learning resources over the course of a given day as well as any problems encountered during this time, the efforts that the student made to solve them, and the solutions that the individual developed. These examples are merely illustrative of what might be recorded in such journals. Notably, these journals can help students document what they have learned while simultaneously helping them improve their understanding of how and what an individual must learn. This approach makes learners more responsible and proactive during the learning process, as they continually evaluate the strategies that they use with the goal of identifying those that are effective and helpful in the learning process (Hill et al. 2020).

In addition, this deliberate and constant process of self-assessment leads to the development of effective strategies that can sustain the learning process while remaining sensitive to emerging learning requirements. *Self-assessment* during the learning process enables learners to remain functional with respect to their achievements and to respond to emerging challenges or opportunities (Hill et al. 2020). The *documentation process* also helps

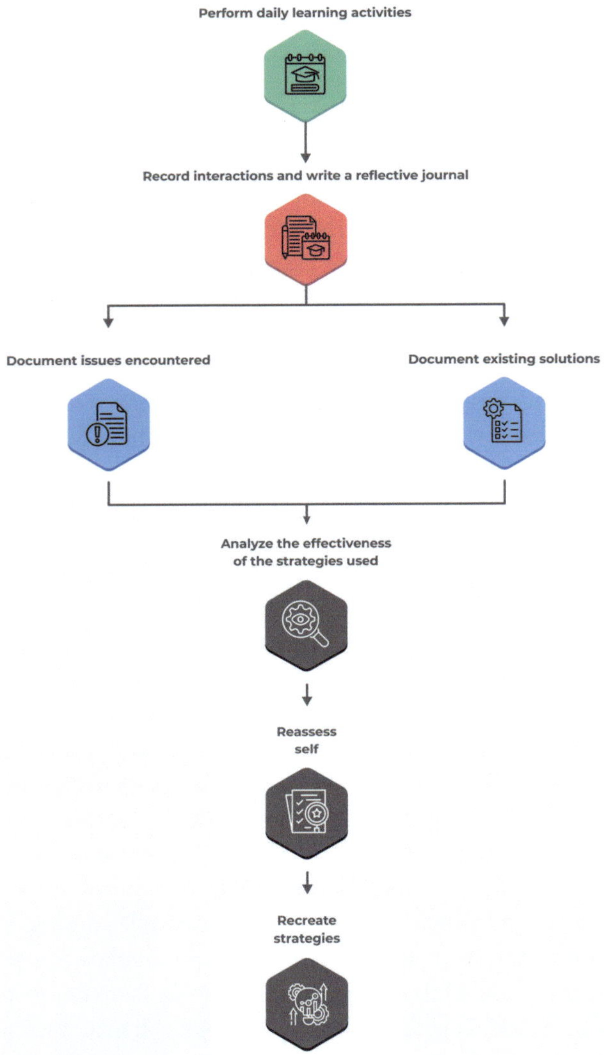

Fig. 7.2 The processes of self-reflection and self-assessment

the learners identify areas that demand change or further development as they consider the patterns that characterize their learning process. This method promotes professionalism within a framework of order and discipline, thereby enabling learners to manage their learning paths independently. Thus, by engaging in consistent self-reflective behaviours, learners can guarantee not only that their educational practices are continuous but also that such practices evolve to ensure a closer match with learners' lifelong goals (Yan and Carless 2021).

Specific tools can be used to accomplish this goal, including the *Self-Directed Learning Readiness Scale 19–22* and the *Oddi Continuing Learning Inventory*, which may be used to assess outcomes (Robinson and Persky 2020).

Table 7.2 Summary of the different types of resources

Type of resources	Frequency of updates	Mode of access	Fields covered
Academic and peer-reviewed journals	Quarterly or annually	Free and subscription-based	Multiple disciplines depending on the scope of the specific journal
Professional forums (i.e., LinkedIn)	Daily	Free and subscription-based	Specific to a given industry or field
Conferences and workshops	Twice per year or annually	Free with registration	Multiple disciplines
Online communities	Daily	Free	Any

7.3.6 Remaining Up-to-Date with the Most Recent Knowledge

Table 7.2 indicates that remaining up-to-date with the most recent developments can ensure relevance and continual growth in one's field. In the rapidly evolving context of nearly every discipline, self-directed learners must employ various strategies to remain informed of new information and trends. For example, it is now possible to read the top academic and peer-reviewed journals, participate in online communities, and attend conferences and workshops with the goal of remaining up-to-date. These activities make it possible for learners to keep pace with developments in their areas of practice and thus to acquire new knowledge and practices in a way that can influence their proficiency and awareness (Alsayer 2023; Mlambo et al. 2021; Zenni and Turner 2021). Additionally, connections with various professions can be more informative and cutting-edge sources than can be obtained through conventional channels. LinkedIn and similar forums or even specific professional interest groups can facilitate discussion, resource sharing, and collaboration, thus rendering the learning process continuous. Continuous interaction with new information and knowledge expands learners' education and increases their flexibility and employability in the workplace (Davis et al. 2020). By engaging with these networks, learners can share knowledge, solve issues in group contexts, and discuss newly developed strategies or opportunities that can be used to enhance their education and future careers.

7.3.7 Take-Home Messages

The strategies outlined in this chapter represent a package that can be identified as a robust framework that learners can use to seize control of their learning processes. Self-direction is central in contemporary learning environments; hence, this chapter is a treasure trove of techniques and approaches pertaining to the task of self-improvement. These tools include the establishment of SMART objectives, the formulation of a well-coordinated study timetable, the use of a variety of resources, the provision of feedback, and the documented habits of self-reflection and self-assessment. Each such tool can help cultivate learners who are proactive, self-directed, and sensitive to change. It is also crucial to ensure that these learners can empower themselves in the same ways, thus guiding their social, personal, and professional endeavours and enabling them to respond to the dynamics of society, which are undergoing dramatic transformations.

In the future, all these skills can be expanded and used to develop advanced self-learning methods within specific disciplines. This insight leads to the next chapter, which focuses on a more specific exploration of the ways in which these general principles may be implemented in specific subject fields and training. We demonstrate how self-directed learning activities result in profound accomplishments and discoveries in various fields by analysing cases and examples drawn from different fields and discussing the scenarios in which they can be applied. This exploration helps improve the learner's repertoire, thus facilitating the acquisition of the subtle techniques that are necessary for learners' efforts to cope with complicated and specific learning environments.

7.4 Summary

In this analysis of SDL, we highlight essential approaches that support the learners' efforts to obtain a full understanding of and take control over the educational process. This analysis of ways of setting accurate learning goals and objectives and constructing detailed learning schedules with regard to a variety of sources and activities, feedback, and reflections reveals that *SDL* can prepare learners to achieve the goal of effective, flexible, and lifelong learning. These methodologies are also conducive to information acquisition and retention and can improve the learner's ability to apply such knowledge in practice. *SDL* has been practised for some time, and it has been demonstrated to enhance various aspects of learners, such as motivation, adaptability in response to complex problems, and the ability to address problems both in and outside the classroom, which represent the keys to success in examinations as well as their future professions.

The tasks of exploring the conceptual meanings of these findings with respect to policy and practice and communicating those meanings to relevant stakeholders are highly important. Learners, educational institutions, and policymakers can adopt and incorporate *SDL* principles into their curricula and learning spaces with the aim of promoting self-directedness among learners. This task may include the implementation of more customized learning solutions, efforts to ensure that the available learning resources are more diverse, and regular and efficient feedback sessions. The positive effects of *SDL* in the workplace can promote creativity and flexibility within the working environment. Employers can support *SDL* by facilitating continuous professional development and enhancing the organization's learning culture. Finally, in line with the established principles of *SDL*, not only the programmes used in educational systems and workplaces but also individual members of societies can improve their effectiveness and prepare for further transformations in the newly emerging world, which is rapidly becoming more complicated.

References

Alsayer AA. Learners' experiences in an online learning environment: an analysis of the impact of international collaboration. SAGE Open. 2023;13:21582440231208524.

Bürgermeister A, Glogger-Frey I, Saalbach H. Supporting peer feedback on learning strategies: effects on self-efficacy and feedback quality. Psychol Learn Teach. 2021;20:383–404.

Burgess A, Van Diggele C, Roberts C, Mellis C. Feedback in the clinical setting. BMC Med Educ. 2020;20:460.

Chatterjee D, Corral J. How to write well-defined learning objectives. J Educ Perioper Med. 2017;19:E610.

Davis J, Wolff HG, Forret ML, Sullivan SE. Networking via LinkedIn: an examination of usage and career benefits. J Vocat Behav. 2020;118:103396.

Gilakjani AP. Visual, auditory, kinaesthetic learning styles and their impacts on English language teaching. J Stud Educ. 2012;2:104.

Henderson M, Phillips M, Ryan T, Boud D, Dawson P, Molloy E, Mahoney P. Conditions that enable effective feedback. High Educ Res Dev. 2019;38:1401–16.

Hill M, Peters M, Salvaggio M, Vinnedge J, Darden A. Implementation and evaluation of a self-directed learning activity for first-year medical students. Med Educ Online. 2020;25:1717780.

Larabi-Marie-Sainte S, Jan R, Al-Matouq A, Alabduhadi S. The impact of timetable on student's absences and performance. PLoS One. 2021;16:e0253256.

Loeng S. Self-directed learning: a core concept in adult education. Educ Res Int. 2020;2020:1–12.

Mlambo M, Silén C, McGrath C. Lifelong learning and nurses' continuing professional development, a metasynthesis of the literature. BMC Nurs. 2021;20:62.

Morris TH, Bremner N, Sakata N. Self-directed learning and student-centred learning: a conceptual comparison. Pedagog Cult Soc. 2023:1–20. https://doi.org/10.1080/14681366.2023.2282439.

Nuuyoma V. Feedback in clinical settings: nursing students' perceptions at the district hospital in the southern part of Namibia. Curationis. 2021;44:e1–e12.

Robinson JD, Persky AM. Developing self-directed learners. Am J Pharm Educ. 2020;84:847512.

Vincent-Lancrin S. Fostering and assessing student critical thinking: from theory to teaching practice. Eur J Educ. 2023;58:354–68.

Yan Z, Carless D. Self-assessment is about more than self: the enabling role of feedback literacy. Assess Eval High Educ. 2021;47:1116–28.

Yang L, Chiu MM, Yan Z. The power of teacher feedback in affecting student learning and achievement: insights from students' perspective. Educ Psychol. 2021;41:821–4.

Yen PY, Kellye M, Lopetegui M, Saha A, Loversidge J, Chipps EM, Gallagher-Ford L, Buck J. Nurses' time allocation and multitasking of nursing activities: a time motion study. In: AMIA annual symposium proceedings. Washington, DC: American Medical Informatics Association; 2018. p. 1137–46.

Zenni EA, Turner TL. Planning and presenting workshops that work: a faculty development workshop. MedEdPORTAL. 2021;17:11158.

Mastering Time Management in the Context of Education in the Health Professions

8

Khalid A. Bin Abdulrahman, Abdullah A. Alzayed,
and Ibrahim A. Bin Ahmed

Learning Objectives

1. *Identify effective time management techniques.*
   Learners will be able to recognize and apply key time management strategies, such as prioritization using the Eisenhower matrix, the Pomodoro technique, and the SMART framework for goal setting, to balance academic and personal responsibilities effectively.
2. *Create and implement a structured schedule.*
   Learners will develop the ability to establish a feasible and structured schedule that includes setting clear, actionable goals, minimizing disruptions, and fostering a conducive learning environment to enhance productivity and reduce stress.
3. *Analyse and adapt to challenges in time management.*
   Learners will evaluate common time management challenges, such as procrastination and unforeseen circumstances, and implement adaptive strategies, including ongoing assessment and collaboration, to maintain academic progress and personal well-being.

K. A. Bin Abdulrahman (✉)
Department of Medical Education, College of Medicine, Imam Mohammad Ibn Saud Islamic University (IMSIU), Riyadh, Saudi Arabia
e-mail: kab@imamu.edu.sa

A. A. Alzayed
Department of Pediatrics, College of Medicine, Imam Mohammad Ibn Saud Islamic University (IMSIU), Riyadh, Saudi Arabia
e-mail: aaalzayed@imamu.edu.sa

I. A. Bin Ahmed
Department of Family and Community Medicine and Medical Education, College of Medicine, Imam Mohammad Ibn Saud Islamic University (IMSIU), Riyadh, Saudi Arabia
e-mail: ibinahmed@imamu.edu.sa

K. A. Bin Abdulrahman, H. Darami (eds.), *Essential Learning Skills for Health Professions Students*, https://doi.org/10.1007/978-981-96-5670-7_8

8.1 Introduction

Time management is an essential skill for learners pursuing an education in healthcare, especially for those who study the fields of medicine, dentistry, nursing, pharmacy, and applied health sciences. Balancing rigorous projects with personal responsibilities and hands-on training can be challenging for learners who seek to excel in their studies while living a fulfilling personal life and ensuring sufficient self-care. Therefore, the development of solid approaches to time management can help promote academic success and lay a strong foundation for individuals' careers in the field of healthcare. Mastery of such skills is essential with regard to learners' ability to participate in classes, complete assignments, and prepare for examinations successfully, thereby mitigating the harmful effects of postponement, depression, anxiety, and adverse observations that might otherwise obstruct their ability to advance in the field of healthcare. This chapter explores vital strategies that learners can use to manage their time and priorities effectively, attain academic success, and navigate their educational journeys while facing a minimal level of psychological stress.

8.2 Recognizing the Importance of Time

Recognizing the value of time is crucial for learners in healthcare settings. Research has reported that effective time management allows learners to complete more work in less time because their attention is focused, thus enabling them to avoid wasting time on disruptions (Wolters and Brady 2021). For example, the efficient use of time can decrease stress as learners complete items on their to-do lists. Moreover, time is a limited and priceless resource, and its effective management directly impacts both academic performance and personal safety. In the challenging field of healthcare education, where courses are dense and prospects are high, every second counts. Learners must understand that every second spent on non-essential events entails opportunity costs with respect to their educational and career ambitions.

Learners in the field of healthcare often face a multitude of responsibilities, such as participating in lectures, engaging in clinical rotations, reviewing in preparation for examinations, and completing projects. The sheer volume of such tasks can be devastating; thus, prioritizing and managing one's time professionally are imperative in this context. Acknowledging the significance of time allows learners to allocate their efforts strategically, including by emphasizing activities that contribute most significantly to their goals (Wolters and Brady 2021). This approach not only improves learners' academic performance but also ensures that they can adopt a balanced approach to personal safety, thereby decreasing stress and preventing exhaustion. By acknowledging the importance of time, students can nurture an approach that focuses on resourcefulness and output. This mindset is critical with respect to success in both academic and practical endeavours. In practical terms, this approach involves setting clear, achievable goals and adhering to a structured schedule. For example, a learner might allocate specific hours to the tasks of studying, attending classes, and relaxing, thereby ensuring that every aspect of their life receives appropriate attention.

Moreover, respecting time can facilitate the development of self-discipline and accountability. This approach communicates a sense of firmness and determination, thus encouraging students to make the most of their educational opportunities. This practical structure not only helps students understand sudden academic provisions but also confirms that they are ready to face the fast-paced, time-sensitive situations involved in the healthcare occupation (Terzi et al. 2024). Essentially, recognizing the implications of time focuses on making conscious choices that are in line with one's long-term goals. For students in the field of healthcare, recognizing such standards represents a crucial step in the tasks of understanding their academic goals, ensuring personal safety, and ultimately surpassing their future professions.

8.3 Establishing Objectives and Assignments

Developing strong resolutions represents a substantial step in the process of promoting positive time management skills among healthcare students. In light of the difficult nature of their studies, a distinct purpose can help such students remain steady in response to stress and can confirm that hard work is associated with lasting ambitions. Students should set goals on a "quarterly, monthly, weekly, and daily basis by means of the SMART principles that comprises Specific, Measurable, Achievable, Relevant, and Time-bound" (Wilson et al. 2021). Dividing large projects into smaller projects renders these tasks easy to accomplish and facilitates accurate assessments of what can be achieved in a specified time frame.

For example, previous researchers have reported that quarterly goals for a healthcare student can represent a vital project for research. These goals are specific (e.g. completing a research project), measurable (e.g. producing a project report), achievable (i.e. within the given time frame), relevant (e.g. by contributing to educational provisions), and time-bound (e.g. with regard to projects that must be completed by the end of the quarter) (Wilson et al. 2021). Dividing such long-term purposes into smaller, controllable projects can make the task of working on these tasks less overwhelming and more organized.

Monthly goals might emphasize reviewing material for a specific set of examinations or understanding certain medical measures. Weekly goals might include completing an assigned chapter of a textbook, engaging in group study sessions, and preparing for laboratory sessions (Çingöl and Karakaş 2023). A well-structured weekly schedule that includes class sessions, study sessions, self-care activities, and individual commitments offers a clear overview of the individual's time, thus facilitating better planning and enabling the available hours to be used more effectively. Constant updates and refinements to such schedules can help improve the allocation of time.

The articulation of such goals can help learners maintain their attention and ensure that their diligent work is in line with their continued motivation. Every goal should be defined clearly and broken down into actionable steps (Çingöl and Karakaş 2023). This approach not only makes it easier for individuals to track their progress but also elicits a sense of achievement because every task has been completed. Through constant assessments and reviews of such goals, learners can establish a coherent schedule or emphasis, thereby ensuring that they make continuous progress towards their primary goals.

8.4 Distinguishing Priorities

Learners in the field of healthcare should develop the ability to distinguish between significant or urgent priorities and irrelevant or pressing projects. Use of the Eisenhower matrix represents an ideal strategy for achieving this goal (Kennedy and Porter 2022). This matrix categorizes tasks into the following four quadrants on the basis of their urgency and significance:

1. *Important and Urgent*: This category involves projects that require immediate attention and are critical to long-term goals.
2. *Important but Not Urgent*: This category includes projects that are vital with respect to long-term success but do not require instant action.
3. *Not Important but Urgent*: This category pertains to projects that require instant consideration but do not contribute substantially to long-term goals.
4. *Not Important and Not Urgent*: This category involves projects that are neither time-sensitive nor critical to long-term success.

Projects in quadrant 1 require immediate attention and are significant with regard to long-term goals. Among learners in the field of healthcare, such tasks might include studying for an upcoming major examination, preparing for a clinical skills test, or submitting a critical task whose deadline lies in the near future (Kennedy and Porter 2022). An emphasis on such tasks ensures that crucial deadlines are met and that vital knowledge can be acquired. Tasks in quadrant 2 are crucial with regard to lasting success but do not require instant action. For example, students might engage in regular exercise, review their lecture notes consistently, and work on long-term research projects. In this case, scheduling time for such activities can prevent them from becoming urgent crises later and support students' general academic and personal safety.

The projects in quadrant 3 mostly include interruptions that demand instant attention but do not necessarily contribute to long-term goals. For example, a student might engage in optional meetings, answer nonurgent emails, or address minor administrative issues (Wilson et al. 2021). The delegation of such tasks or the establishment of precise times for addressing them might prevent these issues from diverting students from more critical work. Projects in the final quadrant are mostly time-wasters and should be reduced or eliminated. For example, excessive use of social media browsing, unproductive discussions, or binge-watching TV shows can be limited or eliminated. Understanding and limiting such activities can ensure that more crucial time is available for important and urgent projects.

The consistent application of the Eisenhower matrix can enable learners in the field of healthcare to prioritize their projects successfully. For example, if a learner faces an upcoming pharmacological examination (quadrant 1), they must emphasize the task of studying for that examination before they work on any other, less important projects, including excessive social media use (quadrant 4) (Wilson et al. 2021). However, students should work regularly on prolonged tasks, such as research papers that are due the following month (quadrant 2), to prevent last-minute stress. Such prioritization helps prevent the accumulation of insignificant projects that place demands on students' precious time and energy.

Table 8.1 presents a simplified priority table with examples that students can use to manage their study time effectively.

Table 8.1 A simplified *priority table* with examples that students can use to manage their study time effectively

Priority table for time management			
Priority	Action	Example	What to do
High importance, high urgency	Do it immediately	Preparing for an exam tomorrow Submitting an assignment due today	Focus on these tasks first and complete them as soon as possible
High importance, low urgency	Plan to do it	Reviewing notes for finals in 2 weeks Researching for a long-term project	Schedule these tasks into your calendar to work on them gradually
Low importance, high urgency	Delegate or minimize	Replying to a non-essential email Completing a quick survey	Complete these tasks quickly or delegate if possible
Low importance, low urgency	Eliminate or postpone	Scrolling through social media Watching random YouTube videos	Limit time on these tasks or avoid them when studying

This method is inspired by the Eisenhower matrix, which categorizes tasks based on urgency and importance

Steps for students who want to use the priority table:

1. *List all tasks* you need to do (assignments, exams, extracurriculars, etc.)
2. *Categorize each task* based on the priority table
3. *Focus on the top-left quadrant* (important and urgent) tasks first
4. *Plan your study sessions* around important but less urgent tasks to avoid last-minute stress

Illustrative Example

Suppose you have:

- Human anatomy test tomorrow (*High Importance, High Urgency*) → Study first
- Host defence test due in 5 days (*High Importance, Low Urgency*) → Plan to write 200 words daily
- Group project meeting in 2 hours (*Low Importance, High Urgency*) → Attend briefly and focus on essentials
- Old friends social meeting (*Low Importance, Low Urgency*) → Attend during free time, not study time

This approach ensures that your *critical deadlines* are met, and you steadily progress towards long-term goals while avoiding distractions

8.5 Establishing a Conducive Environment

Learners in the field of healthcare, who face demanding and rigorous academic schedules, require a conducive environment to ensure that they can manage their time effectively. Research has revealed that a discretionary study setting increases learners' attentiveness, prevents distractions, and enhances their productivity, thus allowing students to manage their time more successfully and leading to better educational results (Mash and Edwards 2020).

A conducive setting for students can include several elements, including a quiet and organized space in which students can study, the necessary resources, reliable study practices, tools for organization, and personalization and relief. For example, a quiet and prepared space for learning should be free of any disruptions, such as visual clutter, loudness, and regular interruptions (Mash and Edwards 2020). A good location for study includes a comfortable chair, a steady desk or table that receives sufficient lighting, and access to all vital study resources. Tidy and organized spaces can limit students' anxiety and help them maintain their focus, thus making it easier for students to complete the assigned tasks.

Furthermore, the development of reliable learning practices is vital because such practices can elicit a sense of structure and respect, thus ensuring that students can effortlessly assign particular times to learning, project work, and course participation. For example, dedicating some number of hours each day to the task of studying can enable students to develop a routine that can increase their efficiency (Mash and Edwards 2020). Regular breaks can also be used to prevent exhaustion among students and their preserve mental acuity. Various organizational tools, such as digital calendars, designers, and project management apps, can be used to establish such a favourable study setting. Such tools can help students keep track of their plans, set reminders regarding vital deadlines, and plan their learning sessions effectively. For example, students can employ a digital calendar to divide their learning time, set aside time for breaks, and develop strategic plans for examinations and other forms of progress.

The idea that students can personalize their learning spaces to ensure that those spaces are in line with their own predilections might also represent an important way of establishing a satisfactory setting. Some students might view circumstantial music or ambient noise as important, whereas others may prefer complete silence. Ensuring that one's learning space is comfortable and features an appropriate ergonomic arrangement can limit physical anguish and support continual learning sessions (Mash and Edwards 2020). Through such methods, learners in the field of healthcare can successfully improve their time management skills and proficiency, thereby enabling them to attain success in their classes and improving their general safety.

8.6 Minimizing Disruptions

In most cases, students who engage in various disruptions and pointless, time-consuming activities while studying, especially in the field of healthcare, face significant challenges and problems in terms of academic achievement (Pellegrino et al. 2022). The best strategy that can be used to address such problems is to encourage students first to identify common disruptions, such as binge-watching and social media use. This approach allows students to select a significant method that can be used to address the problem. They can use the Pomodoro technique to categorize and prevent disruptions (Pellegrino et al. 2022). This practice involves working for a set time of approximately 25 minutes, followed by a short break of approximately 5 minutes. This technique helps students maintain their attention and prevent burnout by encouraging them to take methodical breaks while continuing to engage in productive study sessions. For example, a student might employ a timer app to implement this method, thus allowing them to maintain their full attention during each Pomodoro session while refreshing themselves during breaks.

Moreover, awareness of the use of media platforms and other online disruptions is vital for healthcare learners. These individuals can use online apps or online tools to limit their access to redundant feeds on social media. For example, they can adjust features such as the "Do Not Disturb" function on their devices to prevent distractions. Scholars have proposed that mandating clear limitations with regard to one's friends and family and informing them of the time that one has set aside for study represent important ways of ensuring that those others respect students' schedules (Pellegrino et al. 2022). This time must be communicated at an early point to ensure that these others are prepared to respect that time, thus preventing any confusion or disturbances that could arise as a result of misunderstandings.

8.7 Developing a Feasible Strategy

Students are required to develop an honest and clear plan with regard to their everyday practices or endeavours. This goal can be achieved by breaking larger tasks down into smaller tasks, thus improving the manageability of such work and allow an exact time to be assigned to every action. Such practices might help learners achieve their academic goals by preventing various challenges related to time management. For example, if a student must work on a major study paper that is due in 1 month, they might divide this project into smaller steps, including investigating the topic, generating an outline, writing the different segments of the paper, and reviewing the draft (Koka et al. 2021). Each such smaller project can then be assigned a certain deadline, thus making the project as a whole more manageable.

Assigning specific times to distinct activities can ensure that all essential projects are addressed systematically. For example, a learner might specify that morning hours are dedicated to attending lectures, afternoon hours are dedicated to studying and completing

Table 8.2 An example of weekly study schedule

Weekdays	Activity description
Day 1	Review lecture notes and identify key ideas
Day 2	Review lecture notes and identify key ideas
Day 3	Review lecture notes and identify key ideas
Day 4	Complete practice issues and case studies
Day 5	Engage in a study group discussion
Day 6	Participate in a practice examination and review incorrect answers
Day 7	Rest and light review

given tasks, and evenings are dedicated to extracurricular activities or relaxation (Koka et al. 2021). Developing a daily plan that includes time for every relevant activity enables learners to balance their academic lives with their personal lives more successfully.

8.7.1 Example Strategy

A healthcare student has established a weekly goal of preparing for an upcoming examination. This student might divide their study schedule as follows:

By employing such a strategy consistently, learners can make steady progress towards their goals, thus preventing them from becoming overwhelmed. Table 8.2 demonstrates an example of weekly study schedule.

8.8 Ongoing Assessment and Quantification of Progress

Consistent assessments of the schedule and quantification of every step taken in this context is crucial with regard to effective time management. Learners should periodically analyse their plans and goals to ensure that they remain on track. These analyses may include weekly reflections on what has been discussed and whether adjustments to the plan are necessary. For example, a learner might set aside Sunday evenings specifically to engage in a review session. During such a session, they might assess their progress towards their weekly goal, including by highlighting the results of study sessions and identifying any problems they encountered (Çingöl and Karakaş 2023). When learners observe that they have consistently struggled to master a certain topic, they might alter their plans to include more review sessions pertaining to that specific area for an upcoming week. Tracking one's progress in such a manner ensures that healthcare students can identify areas for improvement, thus eliciting a sense of success. Such continuing reflection can increase learners' inspiration and help them remain dedicated to their goals, thereby ensuring that that they make constant progress and promoting effective time management.

8.9 Developing Self-Esteem Through Accomplishment

Achieving set goals and successfully managing one's time can improve a learner's self-esteem. Every achievement, regardless of its size, elicits a sense of aptitude and assurance. For example, a learner who positively completes 1 week in compliance with their study plan, such as by attending all lectures, completing tasks, and engaging with a study group, is likely to feel a sense of achievement (Çingöl and Karakaş 2023). Such constructive fortification can enable learners to complete more thought-provoking tasks, such as preparing for difficult examinations or working on multifaceted research projects. This kind of positive cycle, which involves setting goals, achieving them, and building confidence, helps learners improve their time management skills. As time progresses, such small successes allow the learner to develop a strong foundation of self-assuredness. This increase in self-esteem is highly valuable with respect to both academic and professional searches, as it can cultivate resilience and a proactive attitude towards future challenges.

8.10 Overcoming Challenges Pertaining to Time Management

Regardless of how diligently they work, learners continue to face significant challenges with regard to managing their time. Common challenges in this context include surprising circumstances (such as disease or individual crises), postponement, and a lack of motivation. Addressing such problems requires a practical and adaptable approach. Research has identified a flexible mindset as significant in this context (Lombardo et al. 2023). Students must be ready to modify their strategies as needed when unforeseen events occur. For example, if a learner becomes sick and cannot continue to adhere to their study plan, they can modify their timetable to recover at a later point, thus confirming that they are on track and preventing them from becoming overwhelmed.

Furthermore, seeking support from counsellors, proficient therapists, or peers might provide learners with substantial direction and motivation during difficult times. For example, if a student experiences stress as a result of delays, they might join a study group in which associates hold each other accountable for completing projects (Lombardo et al. 2023). Counsellors can also propose methods that can be used to promote motivation and time management, and qualified therapists can help learners address fundamental issues such as stress or anxiety.

For example, consider a student who encounters a particular emergency that affects their learning. By collaborating with teachers and asking for extensions for projects, learners might correct their timelines without affecting the quality of their work (Lombardo et al. 2023). This adaptability can ensure that learners have the ability to comply with the demanding procedures for which healthcare students are responsible at both the personal and professional levels.

8.11 Summary

The issue of time management in the context of healthcare education is crucial, and it requires learners to use significant strategies that can help them manage their time. Accordingly, healthcare students should recognize that time management and significant management skills are required by learners in the field healthcare because these factors can help such learners address the demanding aspects of healthcare as well as the thought-provoking academic and clinical tasks for which they are responsible. Therefore, when students in the field of healthcare understand such explicit strategies, including limiting interruptions and overcoming challenges, they can address the demands of their education and ensure their own safety more effectively.

References

Çingöl N, Karakaş M. Effect of the management in nursing course on students' time management and career planning attitudes: a single-group pre-test post-test study. Nurse Educ Today. 2023;125:105797.

Kennedy DR, Porter AL. The illusion of urgency. Am J Pharm Educ. 2022;86:8914.

Koka R, Koka R, Skadiņš I. Time management experience for 1st year students of the faculty of medicine. Eur J Nat Sci Med. 2021;4:81–94.

Lombardo L, Ehlers J, Lutz G. Mindset and reflection-how to sustainably improve intra- and interpersonal competences in medical education. Healthcare (Basel, Switzerland). 2023;11:859.

Mash B, Edwards J. Creating a learning environment in your practice or facility. S Afr Fam Pract. 2020;62:e1–5.

Pellegrino A, Stasi A, Bhatiasevi V. Research trends in social media addiction and problematic social media use: a bibliometric analysis. Front Psych. 2022;13:1017506.

Terzi E, Isik U, Inan BC, Akyildiz C, Ustun UD. University students' free time management and quality of life: the mediating role of leisure satisfaction. BMC Psychol. 2024;12:239.

Wilson R, Joiner K, Abbasi A. Improving students' performance with time management skills. J Univ Teach Learn Pract. 2021;18:16.

Wolters CA, Brady AC. College students' time management: a self-regulated learning perspective. Educ Psychol Rev. 2021;33:1319–51.

Critical and Creative Thinking in the Context of Education in the Health Professions

9

Khalid A. Bin Abdulrahman, Fahad A. Alateeq, and Imran Siddiqui

Learning Objectives

1. *Analyse the role of critical thinking in medical education.*
   Students will be able to evaluate how critical thinking enhances clinical decision-making, reduces medical errors, and promotes self-directed learning in the context of healthcare.
2. *Demonstrate the importance of creative thinking in addressing healthcare challenges.*
   Students will develop the ability to apply creative thinking strategies to solve complex, real-world problems, including adapting to dynamic healthcare environments and novel crises like pandemics.
3. *Apply educational strategies to foster critical and creative thinking.*
   Students will learn to utilize and assess teaching methods such as problem-based learning (PBL), case-based learning (CBL), and flipped classroom techniques to enhance critical and creative thinking skills in medical education.

K. A. Bin Abdulrahman (✉)
Department of Medical Education, College of Medicine, Imam Mohammad Ibn Saud Islamic University (IMSIU), Riyadh, Saudi Arabia
e-mail: kab@imamu.edu.sa

F. A. Alateeq
Department of Family and Community Medicine and Medical Education, College of Medicine, Imam Mohammad Ibn Saud Islamic University (IMSIU), Riyadh, Saudi Arabia
e-mail: faateeq@imamu.edu.sa

I. Siddiqui
Department of Medical Education, Burnett School of Medicine at TCU, Fort Worth, TX, USA
e-mail: i.siddiqui@tcu.edu

K. A. Bin Abdulrahman, H. Darami (eds.), *Essential Learning Skills for Health Professions Students*, https://doi.org/10.1007/978-981-96-5670-7_9

9.1 Introduction

Education in the medical and health professions plays an instrumental role in the task of preparing future personnel and leaders in the field of healthcare. Given the significance of this sector with regard to efforts to promote public health, education in the medical and health professions must be designed to promote effective learning. The incorporation of critical and creative thinking into the curricula used in this context is key to the task of ensuring that students are prepared to address both existing and emerging challenges in the twenty-first-century healthcare environment. This chapter explores the meaning of critical and creative thinking in the context of education in the medical and health professions, highlights the importance of such education for students in the medical and health sciences, and discusses strategies that can be used to promote these skills.

9.2 The Meaning of Critical and Creative Thinking in the Context of Medical Education

Critical thinking refers to the ability to identify and assess issues and examine relevant pieces of information to reach an appropriate conclusion (Kaur and Mahajan 2023). As noted by Zayapragassarazan et al. (2016), critical thinking is characterized by the ability to search for and identify flaws in arguments and reject claims that lack supporting evidence. In the context of medical education, critical thinking helps students examine their learning needs and understand their perspectives, which can help improve their clinical decision-making and problem-solving abilities (Kaur and Mahajan 2023). Given that critical thinking can help students identify their learning needs, it plays a role in the task of promoting self-directed learning.

Critical thinking in the context of medical education can be *humanist*, *biomedical*, or *social justice-oriented* (Kahlke and Eva 2018). *Humanist critical thinking* focuses on social good and seeks to promote positive relationships among human beings. This approach stands in contrast to *biomedical critical thinking*, which is virtually synonymous with critical reasoning (Kahlke and Eva 2018). From this perspective, critical thinking emphasizes logic and rationality but views emotions as a hindrance. Finally, *social justice-oriented thinking* focuses on examining the biases and assumptions that underlie the world (Kahlke and Eva 2018). In this case, an understanding of the social system is important with respect to the ability to think critically. These three perspectives on critical thinking correspond to the notions of humanist, technical, and emancipatory critical thinking highlighted by Kahlke and White (2013) (Fig. 9.1).

Understanding these conceptions of critical thinking is integral with regard to the ability to negotiate the practices and values of different communities within the healthcare environment.

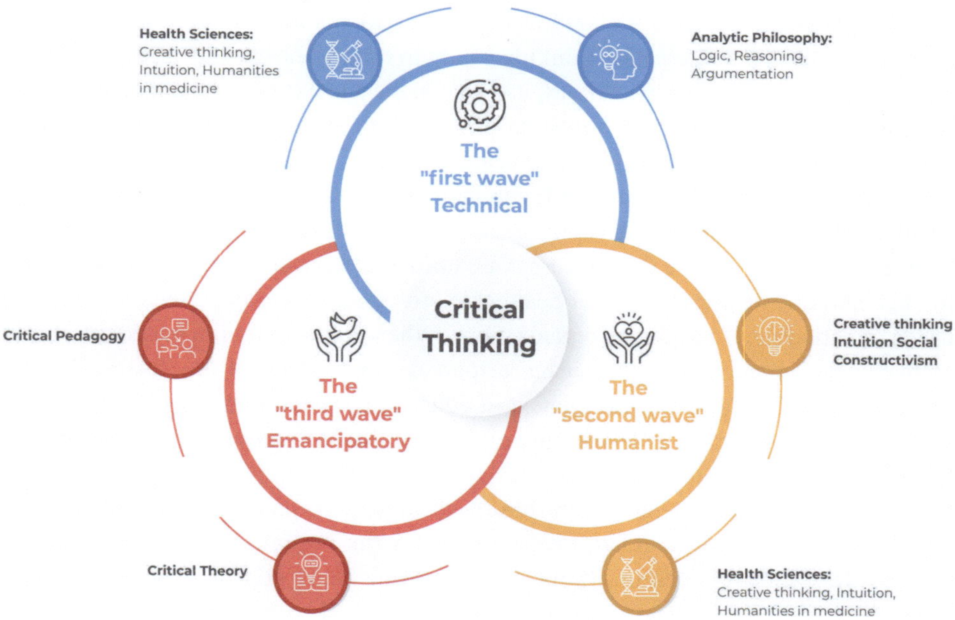

Fig. 9.1 Perspectives on critical thinking. (Source: Kahlke and White (2013))

Creative thinking refers to the ability to consider existing problems from new perspectives. In the context of medical education, creative thinking drives students to employ new approaches to resolve thought–process conflicts (Yelavarthi 2022). Creative thinking is characterized by various key aspects, including the *cognizance of new ideas* and *cognitive flexibility* (Munir and Awan 2022). In light of the complexity of the modern healthcare environment, creative thinking is a necessary component of education in the health professions.

9.3 The Importance of Critical and Creative Thinking for Medical Students

9.3.1 Critical Thinking

Critical thinking skills are necessary with respect to medical students' efforts to navigate the challenges entailed by the modern healthcare environment. According to Shakurnia et al. (2021), critical thinking among healthcare professionals is associated with improved patient and health outcomes. Namely, critical thinking helps health professionals avoid clinical/medical errors and identify better diagnostic and treatment options for patients (Zayapragassarazan et al. 2016). Importantly, clinical/medical errors are a major problem in the healthcare sector at the global level. Every year,

100,000 patients die, while 400,000 hospitalized patients are injured (Heydarikhayat et al. 2024). Given that creative thinking can help reduce these medical errors, which result in the loss of many human lives, its value in the context of education in the health professions is immense. The cultivation of critical thinking among medical students can help transform the delivery of healthcare.

Critical thinking is also associated with increased productivity and improved understanding of various subjects (Zayapragassarazan et al. 2016). Productivity in the healthcare sector can help ensure that resources are utilized effectively. Improved productivity in the healthcare sector entails that healthcare professionals are better able to meet the needs of patients and healthcare organizations. When productivity improves, the ability of healthcare organizations to manage resources more effectively increases, thereby reducing healthcare costs. In the context of education, critical thinking allows medical students to improve their understanding of different subjects throughout their learning. Essentially, critical thinking enhances the ability of students to acquire valuable knowledge and skills, which can improve the healthcare system. As noted by Kaur and Mahajan (2023), through critical thinking, medical students can become self-directed learners; that is, they can take responsibility for improving their clinical decision-making. Students can develop their problem-solving abilities, which represent a valuable skill for medical practitioners (Kaur and Mahajan 2023). Critical thinking, therefore, has immense value due to its ability to help students improve their understanding of the medical subjects that they study.

Critical thinking also helps medical students improve their confidence and succeed in their careers (Zayapragassarazan et al. 2016). The goal of every medical student is to have a successful career in the healthcare sector. In this sense, confidence is valuable with respect to success in any field. On the basis of critical thinking, students can improve their confidence not only in their work but also in their ability to assess the work of other people. Given that critical thinking helps individuals improve their understanding of different subjects, it can be inferred that a person who exhibits critical thinking skills is confident in their ability to argue for and provide evidence to validate their claims. Even in the context of patient care, such a person is confident in their ability to provide the best possible care to patients. They not only assess patients correctly but also implement procedures accurately. Importantly, critical thinking is associated with reduced clinical/medical errors (Zayapragassarazan et al. 2016). The confidence that the individual gains as a result of learning critical thinking skills is valuable in the healthcare sector and can help individuals have successful careers.

9.3.2 Creative Thinking

Medical students require creative thinking skills to address the complex healthcare environment both at present and in the future. Creative thinking can help healthcare professionals address the challenges they encounter in the healthcare sector. By exhibiting creativity, doctors can address the complex problems that they encounter in practice. In their interactions with patients who exhibit complex issues, doctors must provide personalized and feasible solutions that require multidimensional thinking (Ten Haven et al. 2022). In such situations, doctors must deviate from normal protocols and think outside the box to develop solutions that meet the needs of patients in a given context. In this sense, medical professionals can use creative thinking to identify applicable evidence that they can employ to address the contextual needs of customers. Creative thinking thus equips medical students with important skills and abilities that they need to address challenges in the healthcare sector.

Creative thinking is also important for medical students, as it promotes adaptability and flexibility, which are valuable with regard to care provision. The rapidly changing healthcare environment demands creativity, given that medical professionals are expected to react flexibly to new and complex problems (Ten Haven et al. 2022). A specific example of such a challenge in the field of healthcare that demands creative thinking is the COVID-19 pandemic. According to Munir and Awan (2022), during the COVID-19 pandemic, creative thinking was a necessary tool with respect to healthcare professionals' efforts to understand, diagnose, and treat diseases. When the healthcare sector faces novel challenges such as COVID-19, medical professionals must think creatively to identify feasible solutions. Given their value with regard to efforts to address novel challenges in the healthcare environment, critical thinking skills represent a vital component of learning for medical students.

9.4 Strategies That Can Be Used to Promote Critical and Creative Thinking Among Medical Students

The task of promoting critical and creative thinking in the context of medical education is essential with regard to efforts to prepare medical students to address various challenges in the healthcare sector and improve health outcomes. Medical educators can employ several strategies, including problem-based learning; case-based learning; flipped classroom teaching; reflexive writing; the think, pair, and share strategy; and concept mapping (Zayapragassarazan et al. 2016; Kaur and Mahajan 2023). These strategies are discussed in further detail below.

9.4.1 Problem-Based Learning (PBL)

Problem-based learning (PBL) is an innovative teaching approach in which students are presented with real-life scenarios that enable them to explore a specific topic in further detail (Kaur and Mahajan 2023). While PBL was developed in 1969 by Howard Barrows for McMaster University, it has been widely adopted in medical education worldwide (Neville 2008). This strategy is based on the assumption that when students are exposed continuously to real-life scenarios, they can develop the skills they need to evaluate a patient's problem, identify the nature of the problem, and make the correct decision to manage the situation.

PBL is characterized by particular cognitive attributes that can enhance learning and creativity among students (Neville 2008). The fact that knowledge is acquired in a clinical context according to this approach ensures that students are able to remember it more easily. Furthermore, PBL is characterized by the elaboration of knowledge during learning (Neville 2008). The similarity of context that characterizes PBL also allows students to recall information more effectively. In this sense, PBL exhibits certain key features that make it an effective way of helping students acquire and practice relevant critical and creative thinking skills.

For educators to employ PBL, they must organize students into small groups that often include between eight and ten students (Trullàs et al. 2022). In these groups, students participate in the processes of identifying a problem, defining concepts, brainstorming ideas, researching, and sharing information in subsequent discussion sessions. The work of educators in this context involves helping students stay on track to achieve their learning goals (Trullàs et al. 2022). Interestingly, PBL also involves other learning methods, such as case-based learning (CBL) and team-based learning (TBL).

While PBL exhibits cognitive attributes that support its effectiveness in the context of medical education, Neville (2008) claimed that it places burdens on students' working memory. In this sense, it can be impossible for students to use their working memory to learn while simultaneously solving problems. Furthermore, Neville (2008) noted that the processes of learning and practising medicine differ at the cognitive level. Nonetheless, Trullàs et al. (2022) reported that PBL is more effective with regard to improving students' communication and social skills, self-learning skills, and problem-solving skills than are traditional methods; all of these skills are valuable in the process of provide healthcare.

9.4.2 Case-Based Learning (CBL)

Although CBL can be incorporated into PBL as described above, it can also be employed as an independent strategy to help students develop critical and creative thinking skills. According to McLean (2016), CBL uses authentic clinical cases to link theory with practice. By utilizing inquiry-based learning techniques and applying the knowledge obtained from theory to these cases, students can be prepared effectively to engage in clinical practice. The key benefits associated with this strategy include its ability to promote clinical problem-solving, reasoning, and self-directed learning.

While CBL seems to overlap with PBL, several elements distinguish these approaches. The goal of PBL is to help students solve the problem with which they are presented, whereas CBL positions clinical cases at the centre of learning, thus allowing students to acquire knowledge regarding diagnosis and management (McLean

2016). In addition, CBL tends to involve more advanced studies than does PBL. While students have baseline knowledge before they engage in CBL, information is explored on an ongoing basis in PBL (McLean 2016). Another difference between these two strategies pertains to the role of the learner. In PBL, the learner participates actively in the session and is often expected to ask questions while exploring the topic at hand. On the other hand, while the learner is expected to participate in CBL, students in this context are already prepared and ready to ask several questions that relate directly to the cases at hand (McLean 2016). In PBL, the teacher is expected to provide the students with the focal case and to avoid interfering or offering excessive guidance. In the context of CBL, in addition to providing cases, the teacher guides the discussion to ensure that specific learning goals are achieved. A major advantage of CBL over PBL is that the former promotes deeper learning (McLean 2016). This learning strategy extends beyond providing the correct answers and tends to be characterized by more critical thinking.

9.4.3 Flipped Classroom (FC) Teaching

The notion of flipped classroom (FC) teaching was identified by Kaur and Mahajan (2023) as a strategy that medical educators can use to inculcate critical thinking skills in their students. In the context of FC, students are provided with learning materials prior to the classroom session, which is not reserved for direct instruction (Kaur and Mahajan 2023). Unlike in traditional classrooms, where learning materials are provided in class, in the context of FC, students interact with the learning materials before participating in the classroom sessions.

As reported by Nichat et al. (2023), the provision of materials at an early point in this context allows students first to acquire knowledge independently and then to focus on problem-solving and active discussions during classroom sessions. FC often tends to employ case-based discussions with the goal of helping learners acquire higher-order problem-solving skills (Nichat et al. 2023). The independent acquisition of knowledge by learners before class sessions ensures that they are more prepared to participate in productive discussions. As reported by Nichat et al. (2023), FC not only promotes self-motivation and independent learning among medical students but also equips them with problem-solving skills. FC is thus an important strategy that medical educators can use to enhance the critical and creative thinking skills of their students.

9.4.4 Reflective Writing

Reflective writing is also a key strategy that can be used by medical educators to promote critical and creative thinking among students. Reflective capacity has been identified as a necessary professional competence that can help healthcare personnel address challenges that emerge in the contemporary dynamic healthcare sector (Mann et al. 2009). In this context, a *reflective practitioner* employs reflection to learn and frame complex issues in practice (Mann et al. 2009). Reflective writing can enhance students' learning given that it is connected to deep approaches to studying. As noted by Mann et al. (2009), reflective writing facilitates the explicit integration of the affective aspects of learning.

9.4.5 Think, Pair, and Share (TPS) Strategy

This strategy involves a form of cooperative learning that is characterized by active student involvement in group discussions (Kaur and Mahajan 2023). When this strategy is used, students first critically examine a problem individually during the *think phase* after they are presented with prompts or questions by the instructor. In this phase, the students process the questions at hand, consider how those questions can be answered, and organize their thoughts. In the *pair phase*, students are paired with others to explore their responses, listen to one another, and provide a consensus answer. Finally, in the *share phase*, these student pairs share their responses with the larger group. As reported by Ganatra et al. (2021), the TPS strategy is more effective than traditional lectures with respect to learning and engagement outcomes.

9.4.6 Concept Mapping

Concept mapping is also a key teaching strategy that can be used to enhance students' critical and creative thinking skills. Concept maps are used to illustrate the thought process visually and are integral in efforts to organize knowledge, concepts, and processes (Wilgis and McConnell 2008). Concept maps have been reported to improve not only critical thinking but also clinical decision-making and problem-solving (Wilgis and McConnell 2008). An example of such a concept map in the context of medical education is illustrated in Fig. 9.2.

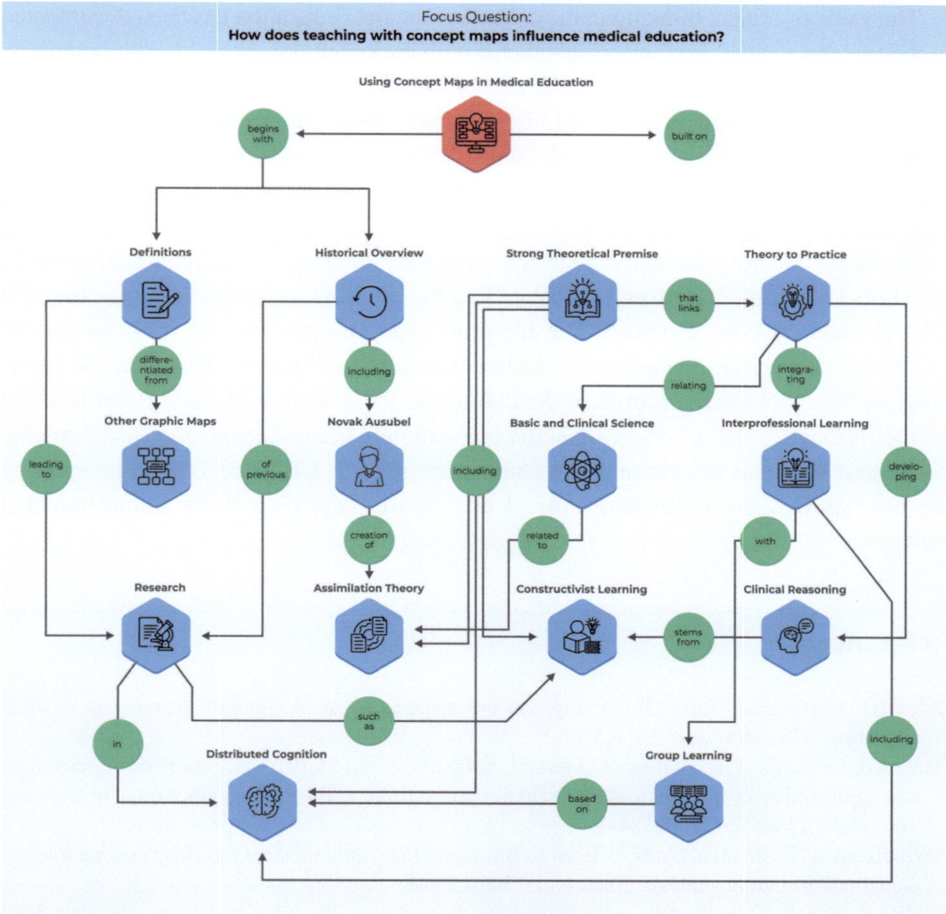

Fig. 9.2 Concept map in the context of medical education. (Source: Daley et al. (2016))

9.5 Summary and Conclusion

Critical and creative thinking skills represent a necessary component of education in the medical professions. The contemporary healthcare environment is rapidly changing, and the incorporation of critical and creative thinking into medical education is essential with respect to efforts to prepare students to face the challenges that they may encounter in practice. Critical thinking is characterized by the ability to examine a problem, find supporting evidence, and draw an informed conclusion. On the other hand, creative thinking helps medical students think in novel ways when they encounter existing problems. Creative thinking skills are thus important with respect to efforts to address various challenges that may emerge in the field of healthcare, such as COVID-19.

The value of critical thinking in the context of medical education has been documented in the literature, which has linked this factor with improved patient and health outcomes. Not only does critical thinking help health professionals prevent medical errors; it also enables them to identify better diagnoses and treatment options for patients. Creative thinking promotes adaptability and flexibility among healthcare professionals; it is thus important with respect to efforts to promote patient-centred care and address emerging challenges in the field of healthcare.

Medical educators can employ several strategies to instil critical and creative thinking skills in their students, such as PBL, CBL, FC teaching, reflective learning, the TPS strategy, and concept mapping. The literature has reported that the most frequently employed strategy in the context of medical education is PBL; furthermore, the popularity of this approach is rooted in the claim that the exposure of students to real-life scenarios enables them to develop skills that can help them manage and treat patients. Given that PBL can incorporate other strategies, such as CBL and TBL, it is arguably the best strategy for cultivating critical and creative thinking skills among medical students.

References

Daley BJ, Durning SJ, Torre DM. Using concept maps to create meaningful learning in medical education. MedEdPublish. 2016;5:19.

Ganatra S, Doblanko T, Rasmussen K, Green J, Kebbe M, Amin M, Perez A. Perceived effectiveness and applicability of think-pair-share including storytelling (TPS-S) to enhance clinical learning. Teach Learn Med. 2021;33:184–95.

Heydarikhayat N, Ghanbarzehi N, Sabagh K. Strategies to prevent medical errors by nursing interns: a qualitative content analysis. BMC Nurs. 2024;23:48.

Kahlke R, Eva K. Constructing critical thinking in health professional education. Perspect Med Educ. 2018;7:156–65.

Kahlke R, White J. Critical thinking in health sciences education: considering “three waves”. Creat Educ. 2013;4:21–9.

Kaur M, Mahajan R. Inculcating critical thinking skills in medical students: ways and means. Int J Appl Basic Med Res. 2023;13:57–8.

Mann K, Gordon J, MacLeod A. Reflection and reflective practice in health professions education: a systematic review. Adv Health Sci Educ. 2009;14:595–621.

McLean SF. Case-based learning and its application in medical and health-care fields: a review of worldwide literature. J Med Educat Curri Develop. 2016;3:JMECD.S20377.

Munir A, Awan OA. Creative thinking: its importance and how to cultivate it. Acad Radiol. 2022;29:1610–2.

Neville AJ. Problem-based learning and medical education forty years on: a review of its effects on knowledge and clinical performance. Med Princ Pract. 2008;18:1–9.

Nichat A, Gajbe U, Bankar NJ, Singh BR, Badge AK. Flipped classrooms in medical education: improving learning outcomes and engaging students in critical thinking skills. Cureus. 2023;15:e48199.

Shakurnia A, Fazelinia T, Khajeali N. The trend of critical thinking disposition in medical students and its relationship with their academic performance. J Educ Health Promot. 2021;10:479.
Ten Haven A, Pragt E, Luijk SJV, Dolmans DHJM, van Mook WNKA. Creativity: a viable and valuable competency in medicine? A qualitative exploratory study. Med Teach. 2022;44:1158–64.
Trullàs JC, Blay C, Sarri E, Pujol R. Effectiveness of problem-based learning methodology in undergraduate medical education: a scoping review. BMC Med Educ. 2022;22:104.
Wilgis M, McConnell J. Concept mapping: an educational strategy to improve graduate nurses' critical thinking skills during a hospital orientation program. J Contin Educ Nurs. 2008;39:119–26.
Yelavarthi R. The need of creative thinking in Indian medical education. Int J Commun Med Public Health. 2022;10:163.
Zayapragassarazan Z, Menon V, Kar SS, Batmanabane G. Understanding critical thinking to create better doctors. J Adv Med Educ Res. 2016;1:9–13.

Search Techniques for Reliable Information in Health Profession Education

10

Khalid A. Bin Abdulrahman, Hassan Ali Alshehri, and Khalid Ibrahim Alhussaini

Learning Objectives

1. *Evaluate information sources.*
   Students will be able to assess the credibility and reliability of various information sources, including peer-reviewed journals, reputable databases, and nonscientific websites, using criteria such as author credentials, publication date, and purpose.
2. *Differentiate source types.*
   Students will understand the distinctions between primary, secondary, and tertiary sources in the health sciences and apply this knowledge to select appropriate resources for research and evidence-based practices.
3. *Apply effective search strategies.*
   Students will employ advanced search techniques, including the use of keywords, boolean operators, and reputable databases (e.g., pubmed, google scholar, and medscape), to locate relevant and credible healthcare information efficiently.

K. A. Bin Abdulrahman (✉)
Department of Medical Education, College of Medicine, Imam Mohammad Ibn Saud Islamic University (IMSIU), Riyadh, Saudi Arabia
e-mail: kab@imamu.edu.sa

H. A. Alshehri
Department of Pediatrics, College of Medicine, Imam Mohammad Ibn Saud Islamic University (IMSIU), Riyadh, Saudi Arabia
e-mail: haalshehri@imamu.edu.sa

K. I. Alhussaini
Department of Medicine, College of Medicine, Imam Mohammad Ibn Saud Islamic University (IMSIU), Riyadh, Saudi Arabia
e-mail: kialhussaini@imamu.edu.sa

K. A. Bin Abdulrahman, H. Darami (eds.), *Essential Learning Skills for Health Professions Students*, https://doi.org/10.1007/978-981-96-5670-7_10

10.1 Introduction

The use of reliable information by healthcare students is important for enhancing research and developing effective solutions to healthcare challenges. As accessibility to the internet has increased, healthcare students can more easily access information from all over the world. However, this easy access to information and the fact that nearly anyone can publish information online mean that students must develop the ability to recognize reliable information. This chapter explores the techniques and strategies that healthcare students can employ to find reliable information.

10.2 Recognizing Reliable Information

A key step in searching for reliable information is finding credible sources. Observing credible sources ensures that students have accurate and trustworthy information to use in their research activities and to bolster their knowledge. However, how does one recognize that a particular source is credible? Prioritizing peer-reviewed journals, reputable databases, and authoritative websites ensures that healthcare students access information that has been evaluated and verified by experts in the healthcare field. The information from these sources is termed scholarly and is considered accurate and trustworthy. According to Stebbins (2015), scholarly sources are authored by a credentialed researcher or professor. Furthermore, a scholarly article is often published in a peer-reviewed journal, which employs blind peer review to rule out research that has been poorly done. The peer-review process (Fig. 10.1) ensures that only credible studies are accepted for publication.

Research papers published in peer-reviewed journals are considered the most credible because of the rigorous peer review process that results in the rejection of poorly conducted or poorly written research. With respect to the reliability of the source pyramid, research papers are at the top, followed by textbooks and reports, generalist books, newspapers and magazines, and, finally, general websites and social media (Fig. 10.2).

The reliability of sources pyramid provides healthcare students with a framework for recognizing reliable sources. By placing each of the sources they encounter on the pyramid, students can use the most reliable sources for their studies and research activities.

Healthcare students can also recognize reliable information by assessing the authors. In most publications, the credentials of the author are provided. It is important for the student to examine any notes about the author and judge whether they have the necessary qualifications to write credible information. Students can also search for the names of the authors in databases and search engines to determine whether they have published other works. A careful examination of sources and their respective authors is integral for determining the sources of information to use.

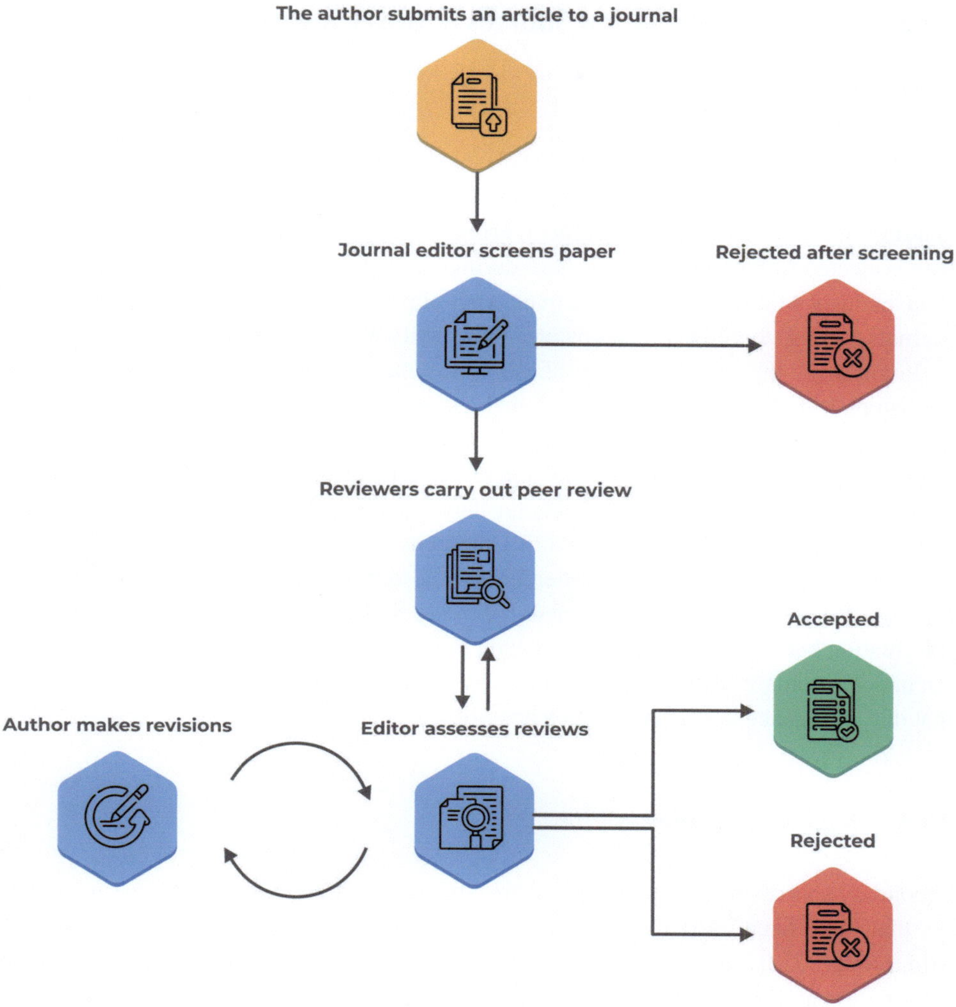

Fig. 10.1 Typical peer-review process. (Source: VoYS (2021))

Fig. 10.2 Reliability of sources pyramid. (Source: The University of Queensland Library (n.d.))

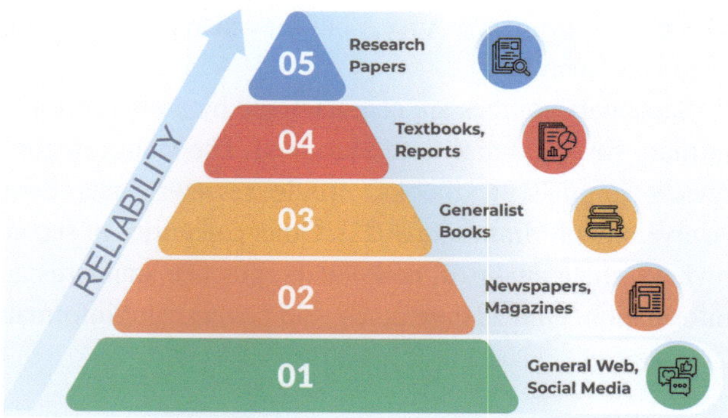

10.3 Types of Information Sources in the Health Sciences

10.3.1 Primary Sources

Primary sources of information in the health sciences provide original results from clinical trials, patient interactions, and experiments. They are records of evidence first discovered and described by healthcare researchers. Primary sources often include the evaluation of data collected in the laboratory or field during experiments designed to test hypotheses (University of Minnesota 2022). The main types of primary sources of information include journals, theses, conferences, and patents (University of Minnesota 2022).

Journals are the main type of publication in which researchers in science report and publish their findings. In this sense, original research, such as experimental studies, clinical trials, and cross-sectional studies, are primary information sources that are published in reputable journals and can be utilized in research by healthcare students. These studies are carried out for the award of an academic degree and are often published later as journal articles (University of Minnesota 2022). Conference papers that report original findings and are presented at professional conferences are also valuable primary sources for healthcare students. Notably, patents on new processes and products are primary sources of information but rarely undergo republication in journals (University of Minnesota 2022). An understanding of these primary sources by healthcare students is imperative to ensure that direct evidence is used in research activities.

10.3.2 Secondary Sources

Secondary sources include publications that examine and discuss original research studies that have been carried out by other researchers. As noted by the University of Minnesota (2022), secondary sources summarize, list, interpret, analyze, and repackage information and data from primary sources. In this case, the aim is to develop new conclusions or update knowledge on the subject (University of Minnesota 2022). Secondary sources synthesize data from several primary sources to provide the audience with a comprehensive review and wider perspective. Not only do they document common findings among primary sources, but they also highlight trends and gaps overlooked by the original research.

Secondary sources are characterized by a reference list that directs the audience to the primary source(s) that were examined. The main categories of secondary sources include review journals, textbooks, article reviews, data compilations, and article indexes (University of Minnesota 2022). Other categories of secondary sources include systematic reviews, meta-analyses, newsletters, practice standards and guidelines, patient education information, clinical care notes, and government information.

While primary research contains the most credible information, secondary sources are also valuable for healthcare students. The analyses, reviews, summaries, and interpretations of primary sources that form the basis of secondary research indicate that healthcare students do not have to undertake the complex and time-consuming task of examining individual primary studies to arrive at a conclusion. In secondary research, such as reviews and textbooks, health information and data are presented in a way that can easily be understood by students and professionals in healthcare. This means that secondary sources save time for students and healthcare professionals.

10.3.3 Tertiary Sources

Tertiary sources are made up of information distilled from primary and secondary sources (the University of Queensland Library n.d.). They provide an introduction or summary of a particular topic and include encyclopedias, fact books, Wikipedia articles, and almanacs (University of Minnesota 2022). Unlike secondary sources that analyze and interpret information, tertiary sources of information do not provide any new information. In addition, tertiary information sources tend to be easily accessible, such as Wikipedia, but note that tertiary sources are not often credited to specific authors. While tertiary sources are at the lower levels of the sources reliability pyramid, they are valuable in providing students with a quick overview of a particular topic. Therefore, they can act as a starting point for research because they contain condensed and easily accessible information from secondary and primary sources. Some tertiary sources also provide references that the student can explore if they would like in-depth information on the topic. Tertiary sources are not appropriate for research and cannot be cited, but they can help students obtain a general overview of a particular topic.

10.4 Efficient Search Techniques

The ability to search for and find relevant and credible sources is integral for health and medical students. Several search techniques can be employed to ensure that an appropriate set of sources are obtained for research purposes. The first technique is to determine the keywords and phrases relevant to the topic. The filler words in a topic can be eliminated to arrive at keywords and phrases (University of Denver 2024). After the keywords and phrases for a topic are identified, synonyms can be determined. This helps in identifying relevant and reliable sources that may have used synonyms or other phrases related to the topic. An important aspect related to keywords is the use of an asterisk (*) in some words, which helps the database retrieve sources with different endings to the word. For instance, the use of an asterisk allows a database to retrieve results for both densities and density (University of Denver 2024).

Table 10.1 A simple table explaining the use of keywords and synonyms tailored for medical students

Term	Explanation	Example
Keywords	Main medical terms related to a topic that help focus on key ideas	*Hypertension, diagnosis, symptoms*
Purpose	Helps you focus your study or research on specific medical concepts	Search "hypertension symptoms" to find relevant resources
Synonyms	Alternative medical or layman terms with the same or similar meanings	*High blood pressure, elevated BP*
Purpose	Helps in understanding diverse terminologies used in exams or practice	A patient might say "high blood pressure" instead of "hypertension"
Combination	Using both keywords and synonyms to prepare comprehensively	Study material titled *Hypertension (High Blood Pressure): Causes & Treatment*

By using *keywords* to grasp core concepts and *synonyms* to understand context and patient communication, medical students can improve both academic and practical understanding

Another important technique related to keywords and phrases is the use of "AND," "OR," and "NOT." These are known as Boolean operators and are integral in helping students refine their search to find relevant sources. As revealed by the University of Denver (2024), three connectors can be employed to narrow or broaden a search. The use of AND in databases narrows the search, allowing for the retrieval of sources containing both terms (University of Denver 2024). OR broadens the search, meaning that the results will be made up of either of the two keywords under research. Finally, NOT narrows down the research but excludes the concepts the student does not want in the search. Another technique that narrows a search is the use of quotation marks. This strategy forces the database to retrieve sources containing the exact phrase within the quotations. For example, a search for "mental health awareness" will exclude results that have "mental health" or "health awareness." This technique can help healthcare students find sources that contain the exact concepts or topics they are exploring. Overall, these techniques allow students to minimize the amount of time needed to find relevant and reliable sources from different databases. Table 10.1 explains the use of keywords and synonyms tailored for medical students.

10.5 Reliable Information on the Web

The internet is vast and contains billions of web pages covering a wide range of information, thus making it difficult to find correct and relevant information. Luckily, several scientific and academic search engines exist that offer reliable sources related to healthcare and medicine. The major reliable search engines that can be utilized include PubMed, Google Scholar, and Medscape.

PubMed is arguably the best search engine and database that students can use to access sources in the biomedical and life sciences fields. The database comprises over

37 million abstracts and literature citations (PubMed 2023). Although the database does not have full-text articles, it provides links to them when they can be found in other sources. A major advantage of PubMed is that the student can access three databases provided by the US National Library of Medicine (NLM): PubMed Central (PMC), MEDLINE, and Bookshelf. PMC contains journal articles that have been selected and reviewed by NLM for archiving, and given that the articles underwent selection and review, the database comprises credible and reliable sources. MEDLINE contains citations of life science articles, whereas Bookshelf contains books, databases, and reports in the healthcare field.

Google Scholar is a valuable search engine that students can use to support their research activities. Not only is it free, but the student can also use it to access academic and gray literature related to healthcare. According to Halevi et al. (2017), Google Scholar offers the advantage of source coverage in the sense that it surpasses the coverage of other scientific literature databases. This is because other databases tend to be controlled; thus, their coverage is selective. In contrast, Google Scholar indexes articles from scientific repositories, publisher websites, and library catalogues. The vast coverage of Google Scholar makes it one of the best search engines for use by health and medical students.

Medscape is an accessible and authoritative database containing sources of clinical information from leading healthcare experts (Medscape 2024). Medscape content is free, and students can access its resources online or through mobile devices. The database comprises over 6000 physician-reviewed articles on diseases and conditions (Medscape 2024). This means that students have, at their disposal, a database that can support answers to clinical questions as well as the diagnosis and treatment of different diseases and conditions. Medscape is also home to over a thousand articles on clinical procedures, which provide detailed instructions for students to learn from and apply (Medscape 2024). With publications on anatomy, drug monographs, and formulary information, Medscape is a valuable database for supporting the research activities of healthcare professionals and students.

These three search engines and databases are not the only resources that students can employ to find relevant healthcare information. Others include Justor, Microsoft Academic, ClinicalTrials.gov, Cochrane, ScienceDirect, Ovid, SpringerLink, Semantic Scholar, Web of Science, and the Wiley Online Library (Gusenbauer and Haddaway 2020). Awareness of these databases is important in facilitating research activities.

For students to search these websites effectively, several tips must be accounted for. First, the filler words in research topics should be removed to obtain appropriate keywords. This allows for specific concepts to be searched, which can yield relevant results. Second, filters such as the range of publication dates, the type of article, and the study design should be used. Third, Boolean operators (AND, OR, and NOT) should be understood and used to narrow down or widen search results.

10.6 Saudi Digital Library (SDL)

The Saudi Digital Library (SDL) is a valuable database for students to access information over a wide range of topics. Established in 2010, the library has more than 240,000 electronic books and is updated regularly (Taala et al. 2019). SDL has partnered with relevant educational organizations and reputable publishers to foster access to resources from all over the world. Examples of publishers that SDL has partnered with include Harvard University, Oxford University Press, Elsevier, Springer, and Taylor & Francis (Taala et al. 2019). With access to materials from these publishers, SDL has emerged as a valuable resource to support the student research activities. For students to access the SDL and the vast resources it offers, they should follow the steps provided by their respective institutions. Typically, student portals contain links that direct them to SDL.

10.7 Reliable or Unreliable Nonscientific Websites

Given that almost anyone can create a website and publish information on the internet, there are numerous websites with health information, some of which are unreliable. While the use of nonscientific websites for medical information is not recommended, some websites can provide general health-related information. It is imperative that a student understands how to evaluate the reliability of websites. In this sense, they must ask themselves key questions, including the following:

Who hosts the website? By examining the hosts/sponsors of websites, students can determine whether the information they publish is reliable. Websites with domain extensions such as .edu, .gov, and .org tend to be more reliable than those with .com extensions.

Who authored and reviewed the information? Through search engines and links provided in the articles, the student can evaluate the credentials of the author(s) and reviewers(s). In this age of the internet, search engines such as Google can provide important information about the authors and reviewers, which can help a student decide whether the authors or reviewers are qualified or have experience writing in a particular field.

When was the information written and published? The healthcare field is characterized by the frequent emergence of new studies, which can invalidate old information. A student need to use up-to-date information when performing research.

What is the purpose of the website? When a website has commercial or promotional interests, there is high risk that it can publish biased and unverified information. A student should access the articles on the website to see whether they promote certain agendas, products, or services.

10.8 Applying Tips in Practice

The search techniques discussed in this chapter are valuable in helping students locate evidence-based information. Not only should students employ keyword search strategies, but they should also use reputable search engines and databases such as Google Scholar, Cochrane, PubMed, and Medscape. The use of Boolean operators in search engines allows students to widen or narrow their searches. This helps students find specific resources in a short time. When possible, students should sift out irrelevant articles in databases by using filters. The use of quotations around key phrases when searching allows students to find resources containing the exact phrase being searched. Subscribing to reputable databases also allows students to access the latest healthcare publications. By employing these techniques, students will not only find relevant and credible resources but also save a significant amount of time.

10.9 Summary and Conclusion

As the internet continues to grow, a vast amount of health information is published online on a daily basis. The ability to assess information sources for relevance, reliability, and credibility is important in fostering evidence-based research and healthcare practices. When searching for resources, peer-reviewed journals, reputable databases, and authoritative websites should be prioritized. Peer-reviewed journal articles are at the top of the credibility pyramid and should be the first type of resource examined. Reputable databases such as PubMed, Google Scholar, and Medscape offer links to scholarly resources that support evidence-based research. Additionally, SDL is a valuable resource for research given that it has partnered with major publishers worldwide.

When searching for information in databases, it is important to identify relevant keywords, synonyms, and phrases that best cover the topic at hand. Boolean operators are valuable in widening or narrowing a search. In addition, understanding the difference among primary, secondary, and tertiary sources can help students discern which resources to use for a quick overview and which resources to use for in-depth research. When assessing websites for health information, the sponsors/hosts of the websites, author credentials, publication dates of the articles, and website purpose should be considered.

References

Gusenbauer M, Haddaway NR. Which academic search systems are suitable for systematic reviews or meta-analyses? Evaluating retrieval qualities of Google Scholar, PubMed, and 26 other resources. Res Synth Methods. 2020;11:181–217.

Halevi G, Moed H, Bar-Ilan J. Suitability of Google Scholar as a source of scientific information and as a source of data for scientific evaluation—review of the literature. J Informet. 2017;11:823–34.

Medscape. Tell me about medscape's clinical database. 2024. https://help.medscape.com/hc/en-us/articles/5019897522061-Tell-me-about-Medscape-s-Clinical-Database.

PubMed. PubMed overview. 2023. https://pubmed.ncbi.nlm.nih.gov/about/.

Stebbins LF. Finding reliable information online: adventures of an information sleuth. Lanham: Rowman & Littlefield; 2015.

Taala W, Franco FB, Sagun RS. Impact of Saudi Digital Library (SDL) to Saudi research output: a review. Open Access Libr J. 2019;6:1–13.

The University of Queensland Library. Health information and research essentials. n.d.. https://uq.pressbooks.pub/health-information-research-essentials.

University of Denver. A guide to health & medical research. 2024. https://libguides.du.edu/health-medical/search-tips.

University of Minnesota. Primary, secondary, and tertiary sources in the health sciences. 2022. https://libguides.umn.edu/c.php?g=986651.

VoYS. Peer review: the nuts and bolts. 2021. https://senseaboutscience.org/wp-content/uploads/2021/09/PEER-REVIEW-the-nuts-and-bolts.pdf.

Effective Presentation and Communication Skills in Health Profession Education

11

Khalid A. Bin Abdulrahman and Hassan Darami

Learning Objectives

1. *Develop presentation skills.*
   Learn to prepare, perform, and reflect on presentations to effectively convey information, engage the audience, and improve professional communication in healthcare settings.
2. *Master effective communication techniques.*
   Understand the principles of clear communication, including active listening, nonverbal cues, and feedback, to enhance patient care and professional collaboration.
3. *Overcome communication barriers.*
   Identify and address common obstacles, such as language challenges, distractions, and time constraints, to ensure successful information exchange in diverse healthcare environments.

K. A. Bin Abdulrahman (✉)
Department of Medical Education, College of Medicine, Imam Mohammad Ibn Saud Islamic University (IMSIU), Riyadh, Saudi Arabia
e-mail: kab@imamu.edu.sa

H. Darami
Department of Obstetrics & Gynecology and Medical Education, College of Medicine, Imam Mohammad Ibn Saud Islamic University (IMSIU), Riyadh, Saudi Arabia

K. A. Bin Abdulrahman, H. Darami (eds.), *Essential Learning Skills for Health Professions Students*, https://doi.org/10.1007/978-981-96-5670-7_11

11.1 Introduction

Effective presentation and communication skills are crucial for healthcare professionals establishing constructive relationships with their patients and improving their health and quality of life. Healthcare professionals in fields such as medicine and nursing must effectively convey information and ideas to coworkers, patients, and other stakeholders within their facility. This chapter explores critical steps for effective presentation, tips for successful presentation, errors to avoid, presentation assessment, the nature and significance of communication, communication flow, and effective communication techniques. Moreover, the essay further explores the common barriers to communication and provides insights for health professionals on how to address them.

11.2 Three Key Steps for Effective Presentation

11.2.1 Prepare

Preparation is key for effective presentation. Thus, health professionals should give themselves plenty of time to prepare thoroughly because a last-minute rush might leave them flustered, especially in delivering the presentation. Research has revealed that this process involves thorough investigation, the logical structuring of information, and the development of a clear and concise outline (Calmer You 2024). These steps ensure that a presenter is well informed about the issue and read to address any concerns that might arise during their presentation.

11.2.2 Perform

The performance skills involved in presenting include the ability to communicate physically and vocally to one's audience. In this case, health professionals should engage their audience through effective eye contact, body language, and vocal variations. Research has shown that body language (which involves what the audience sees) is a significant determination of how passionately individuals can listen to a presentation (Calmer You 2024). Thus, health professionals should build their confidence and professionalism, which are key to developing trustworthiness and keeping the audience's attention.

11.2.3 Reflect

Reflection is key for assessing what went well and will continue, what might have been improved, and what needs to be adjusted in the next presentation. Research shows that reflection after a presentation allows the presenter to assess their performance (Calmer You 2024) and gives them the opportunity to reflect on their experiences of the work as a whole, identify the key learning, and help shape the assessment submissions. The outcome of such activity is key to improving performance. For example, if one was able to make their audience laugh, how did they do that? These reflective aspects determine the effectiveness of upcoming presentations.

11.3 Tips for Successful Presentation

11.3.1 Manage Nervousness and Anxiety

Research has shown that fear of public dialogue is a major form of anxiety (Rolleter 2024) that manifests from minor nervousness to incapacitating fear and panic. Individuals with such fear generally avoid public speaking circumstances or find it difficult to shake hands and have a trembling voice. However, with effective presentation and perseverance, health professionals can overcome this fear. For example, engaging in relaxation techniques and incorporating deep breathing exercises and optimistic self-talk may be helpful for managing this fear that cause nervousness and anxiety. Moreover, practicing one's presentation several times ahead of time builds confidence and averts fear.

11.3.2 Start Strongly

First impressions within a presentation are powerful. Thus, at the start of a presentation, one should seek to capture their audience's attention and ensure that they will not regret being present. Moreover, one can also offer an overview of what is to be discussed in the presentation, learn expectations for the audience, and provide them with good reasons to continue listening (Rolleter 2024). This can be achieved with a brief but compelling opening, showing passion for the subject and developing a connection with the audience from the start.

11.3.3 Focus on the Audience's Needs

A presentation should be built around what the audience expects to learn. If a presenter understands their audience and their expectations, they can easily tailor their presentation to make it more interesting. Thus, health professionals should first take some time to understand who might attend, their expectations, their feelings, and the key message to deliver (Rolleter 2024). Such an initiative might help address the audience's needs and interests. Moreover, understanding their background and expectations helps presenters deliver relevant and engaging content.

11.3.4 Keep It Simple

Research has that audiences find it challenging to follow a presentation that is not developed on simple, clear points (Rolleter 2024). Such a presentation makes it harder for the presenter to deliver their message. Thus, it is important to simplify the message of a presentation to ensure that it is easy to understand. The simple message of a presentation is expected to spread beyond the presenter's sphere of influence. Moreover, making the message simple ensures that the presenter is kept energized every time they need to produce a presentation.

11.3.5 Smile and Make Eye Contact

A simple thing that presenters can do to improve their impact and persuade audiences is to smile and preserve meaningful eye contact with the audience. Positive eye contact is crucial because it helps build rapport with one's audience and keeps them involved in the presentation. Research has shown that deliberating making eye contact with one's audience can communicate how much one cares about their opinions (Rolleter 2024). Moreover, it helps create a connection between speakers and listeners, a bond that is beneficial to both audiences and presenters.

11.3.6 Tell Stories

Stories have been the foundation of human connection since the beginning of human history. Integrating stories within a presentation makes it more applicable and memorable. Research has shown that sharing personal anecdotes or relatable experiences through storytelling helps presenters connect with their audience at a deeper level (Gostin 2022). This emotional connection not only helps build trust with one's audience but also enables presenters to convey their messages genuinely and persuasively.

11.3.7 Use Your Voice Effectively

Presenters need to vary their tone, volume, and pace because this helps preserve their audience's interest and emphasize key points. Spoken words often structure a subject and provide audiences with the opportunity to properly comprehend contexts and follow presentations regardless of complexity (Gostin 2022). Even if a topic is uninteresting, it can be rendered exciting when it is delivered with lively voices, pitch, timbre, speed, and well-placed pauses throughout the presentation.

11.3.8 Use Body Language

Body language says a lot about a presentation and determines its effectiveness. A presenter's body language can reinforce their message and provide audiences with guidance toward the next stage of a presentation. Research has shown that before a presenter even says the first word of a presentation or speech, audiences are more likely to have already

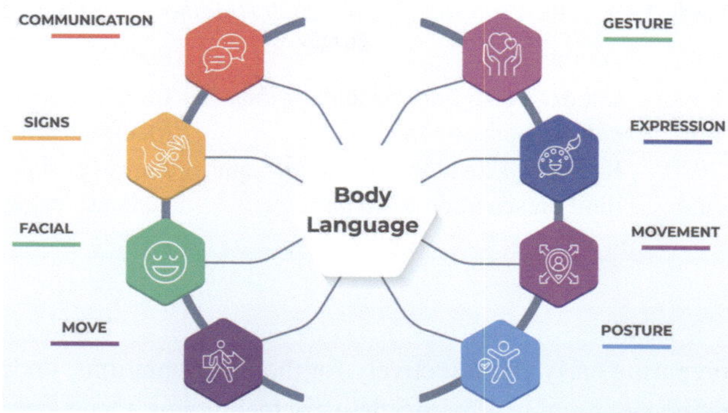

Fig. 11.1 Illustration of body language in a presentation

decided whether they trust them or not (Gostin 2022). Thus, effective body language, including movement and gestures, can reinforce a presenter's message and convey confidence. Figure 11.1 provides an illustration of body language in a presentation.

11.3.9 Remember the 6 × 6 and 2020 Slideshow Rules

According to the 6 × 6 rule, a presenter should include no more than six words per line and no more than six bullet points per slide. The 2020 rule indicates that a presentation should have at most 20 slides, and approximately 20 seconds should be spent on each slide (Gostin 2022). Table 11.1 summarizes the 6 × 6 slideshow rule.

11.3.10 Close with a Take-Home Message and Thank You

The closing remarks of a presentation should clearly demarcate the end. For example, the presenter can use words such as "thank you" that should be spoken, along with a smile and eye contact, instead of merely written on a slide. Moreover, a strong take-home message should be included (Gostin 2022). For example, a medical student can include messages such as "Effective communication and presentation skills are critical in health professions, enabling clear information exchange, enhanced patient care, and improved professional collaboration" (Gostin 2022).

11.4 Avoid Common Presentation Mistakes

Avoiding common mistakes during a presentation is vital to preserving expertise and credibility. Some common mistakes include directly reading from slides, speaking too quickly or softly without pausing, and failing to engage the audience. Avoiding such mistakes is crucial because it helps presenters cement their reputation as good presenters and might even open new doors (Duarte 2020). Health professionals can avoid such errors by

Table 11.1 The *6 × 6 rule* and the *2020 slideshow rule* tailored for health profession students

Rule	Description	Purpose
6 × 6 rule	Use *six words per line* and *six lines per slide* maximum	Ensures concise and readable slides for better focus and retention
2020 rule	Keep text size at least *20 points*, and limit presentation to *20 minutes*	Improves slide readability and maintains audience engagement by avoiding overly long talks

preparing early and effectively for their presentations, understanding their topics, and practicing engaging in effective delivery techniques. Once a presenter eliminates such mistakes, they can automatically look more like a professional presenter and less like a beginner.

11.5 Assess Good and Poor Presentations

Assessing good and poor presentations is crucial for individual and professional growth. Presenters can find effective practices and approaches to integrate into their presentations by observing and examining those of others. A good presentation has various features, such as an interesting hook, audible voice, the use of humor, and a conversational tone (Duarte 2020). However, the bad presentation has no gestures, seems unconfident, is small, has a weak voice, and lacks eye contact. By recognizing and understanding common mistakes, presenters can avoid them in future presentations.

11.5.1 Why Do We Communicate, and What Is Communication?

Effective communication involves exchanging ideas, views, sentiments, facts, and information so that the message is received and comprehended precisely and purposefully. When individuals communicate successfully, both the sender and the receiver feel content. It is crucial in health professions to ensure truthful information sharing, build relationships, and offer effective care (Oliveira 2024). Thus, presenters must speak evidently, preserve an even tone, and make eye contact. When communication is effective, the audience feels pleased and accomplished. Through clear presentation, there is no room for misinterpretation or modification of messages, which reduces the potential for conflict.

11.6 Some Facts About Communication

Communication goes beyond mere words. It includes nonverbal cues such as facial expressions, body language, and gestures that contribute significantly to conveying messages. Active listening and feedback between two parties, specifically the audience and the presenter, are needed for effective communication (Oliveira 2024). Moreover, voice is the most effective form of communication. Listeners hearing samples of an individual's voice can relatively guess whether their presentation will be interesting or boring. Thus, health professionals should be prepared with effective communication skills, mastering all-around facts about communication to ensure that they have a good presentation.

11.7 The Communication Flow

The process of communication involves various steps, from the sender to the response. Effective communication requires a sender, a message, and a recipient, even though the receiver needs to be present or aware of the source's intent to communicate at that specific time. The message can be verbal or nonverbal, or symbolic or written (Fatimayin 2018). It must be in a form that is transmittable and suitable for the channel of communication, whether speech or text. The receiver interprets the message and formulates a response in the form of feedback. This response is communicated back to whoever shared it in the form of a loop. Figure 11.2 provides an illustration of communication flow.

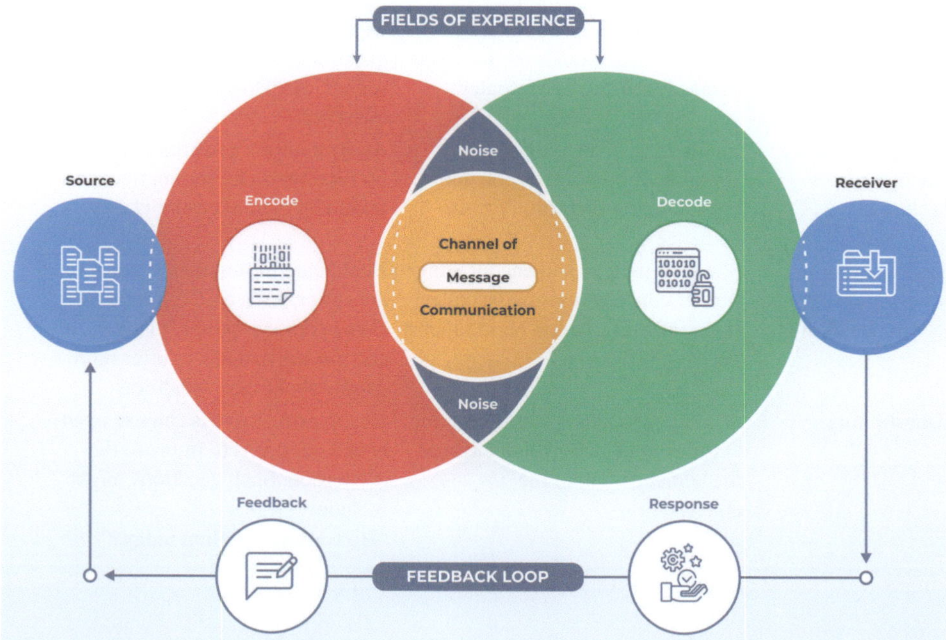

Fig. 11.2 Flow chart illustrating the communication process. The diagram features two overlapping colored circles representing the sender (Source) and the receiver. The left circle is labeled Encode, indicating the sender's process of encoding the message, while the right circle is labeled Decode, representing the receiver's interpretation. At the center of the overlap is the Channel of Message Communication, which is surrounded by Noise, signifying potential interference at various stages. The top of the diagram is framed by Fields of Experience, highlighting how shared background influences communication. Arrows trace the flow of information from source to receiver, supported by icons symbolizing data encoding, decoding, and transmission. A Feedback Loop at the bottom illustrates the dynamic nature of communication, with Response from the receiver feeding back into the sender's next message, ensuring ongoing interaction

11.8 Tips for Effective Communication

Tip	Explanation	Example
Eye contact and visible mouth	Preserving eye contact and ensuring that your mouth is visible help the audience comprehend and connect better	When describing a diagnosis, health professionals should look patients in the eyes to ensure they feel heard and understood
Body language	Positive body language, including open gestures and relaxed posture, strengthens your message and displays confidence	When describing treatment options with patients, health professionals should use open hands and lean forward slightly
Listening skills/ silence	Active listening and the strategic use of silence demonstrate power, self-assurance, and respect for the speaker's contribution	Health professionals should nod and pause after a patient's reply to display that they are considering their words
Smiling face	A pleased face carries openness, accessibility, and honesty, making communication more real	Health professionals can smile while greeting a patient or coworkers to generate a welcoming atmosphere
Checking for understanding	Consistently checking for comprehension helps ensure the audience understands the message being shared by the presenter	After a healthcare professional has explained the procedure, they can ask questions, such as, "Does this make sense?" or "Do you have any questions?"
Summarizing concisely and accurately	Summarizing key points strengthens comprehension and retention of information for the audience	At the end of a consultation, health professionals can summarize the treatment plan to ensure clarity
Encouraging individuals to continue talking	Showing interest and encouraging further conversations helps collect more information and build rapport	Healthcare professionals can ask questions, such as, "Tell me more about your symptoms." This encourages patients to offer more details about their condition
Questioning	Asking questions inspires thinking, clarifies information, and engages the audience within the conversation	Health professionals can use open-ended questions to improve the discussion. Such questions might include "How are you feeling today?"

11.9 Barriers to Communication

Communication can be affected by various factors, including insufficient time, noise, language, and lack of interest, among others. Some of these barriers include the following:

11.9.1 Insufficient Time

Effective time management enables better planning and organization of opinions, ensuring clear and engrossed communication even in highly demanding circumstances such as healthcare fields. However, poor time management can result in timely communication, leading to clearer information, possible misinterpretation, and increased stress among healthcare professionals (Kapur 2018). When presenters feel pressed because of insufficient time, they often need help to convey information in a concise and effective way. Thus, healthcare professionals should plan well, use effective time management tools to avoid confusion, and ensure effectiveness in communication.

11.9.2 Language

Language represents the medium through which every process of communication takes place. This might be verbal (including using words to read, speak, and write) or nonverbal (including facial, sign, and body language) communication. Regardless of such means of communication, health professionals might encounter several barriers related to the inappropriate use of language, such as cultural issues, acronyms, and inappropriate humor, that can lead to misunderstandings between parties (Kapur 2018). Thus, health professionals can decide to learn a foreign language or seek help from interpreters to avoid misunderstandings with patients and other stakeholders.

11.9.3 Noise

Noise can be a crucial barrier preventing an effective communication process between parties. When any form of noise disrupts the process of communication, especially from the sender to the receiver, it might distract the receiver, leading to them not hearing the message properly (Kapur 2018). Noise might also disrupt the sender, making it difficult for them to share the message successfully. Such noise includes physical noise created around the presenter, including a baby crying when they wake up from a nap.

11.9.4 Distractions

Distractions might include background noise, an uncomfortable sitting position, poor lighting, unhygienic rooms, or an environment that might be too hot or cold. Such distractions affect the audience's concentration and, in turn, interfere with effective communication. For example, a responder or audience might be distracted by loud noise (such as a siren, air horn, explosion, or a scream) (Kapur 2018). Such distractions draw the attention of the audience to the source of the noise, limiting their understanding or effectiveness of the communication.

11.9.5 Put-Downs

Negative thinking might leave the presenter nervous and fearful of engaging further in communication. Such events occur when individuals engage in emotional reasoning, which is a critical pattern of negative thinking that often takes the form of trust that if one feels something, it must be true. Moreover, ignoring or failing to react to a comment or an inquiry quickly undermines effective communication (Kapur 2018). Thus, health professionals should work on developing their ability to understand others better by trying to collect information about them, listening to them actively, and imagining how they might feel in their circumstances. Such initiatives might help them address the challenges of put-downs that affect the success of communication.

11.9.6 Lack of Interest

A lack of interest or a wrong attitude can lead to improper communication. When an individual's mind is distracted or preoccupied with other things, they might be unable to form proper messages, listen to what others say, understand the message as needed, and provide proper feedback (Jureddi and Brahmaiah 2016). In this case, communication between them might encounter challenges and need to be more effective. Health professionals should understand such barriers while communicating and trying to modify their ways of communication or messages to ensure that their audiences are back on track and able to concentrate and understand the message.

11.9.7 Discomfort with a Topic

Comfort with a topic can lead to effective communication. For example, some individuals live decisively healthy lifestyles by often exercising and eating only nutritious food but still smoke cigarettes (Jureddi and Brahmaiah 2016). However, healthcare professionals believe that such individuals are selectively overlooking the proof that smoking is unsafe for their health. This selective perception might lead to bias in the communication process between the two parties.

11.9.8 Too Many Questions

Asking an audience too many questions might overwhelm them, leading to ineffective communication. Moreover, too much information might overwhelm the audience (Jureddi and Brahmaiah 2016). Thus, health professionals should use persuasive communication and limit questions to ensure that audiences understand messages without feeling overwhelmed.

In conclusion, healthcare professionals need to present their information clearly so that they can communicate effectively with the audience. Presentation and communication skills not only indicate understanding the topic but also include engaging and connecting with the audience to share the message. By thoroughly preparing, performing confidently, and reflecting on previous presentations and those of others, health professionals can enhance their ability to communicate and address significant barriers to communication. Table 11.2 highlights key barriers to communication along with their descriptions and recommended solutions.

Table 11.2 Key barriers to communication along with their descriptions and recommended solutions

Barrier	Description	Suggested solutions
Insufficient time	Poor time management hinders clear communication and increases stress	Plan ahead, use time management tools, and ensure concise and organized communication
Language	Cultural issues, use of acronyms, and inappropriate humor can cause misunderstandings	Learn foreign languages or use interpreters to bridge communication gaps
Noise	Physical noise disrupts the communication process, leading to distractions for sender/receiver	Minimize background noise and ensure a quiet environment during communication
Distractions	Includes poor lighting, uncomfortable seating, and unhygienic conditions	Create a comfortable and distraction-free environment to maintain audience focus
Put-downs	Negative thinking or ignoring responses undermines communication	Actively listen, empathize with others, and address negative patterns of thinking
Lack of interest	Preoccupied or distracted individuals fail to communicate effectively	Modify messages to re-engage the audience and encourage focus
Discomfort with topic	Bias or selective perception leads to ineffective communication	Address biases by presenting facts neutrally and encouraging open discussions
Too many questions	Overwhelming the audience with excessive questions or information disrupts communication	Limit the number of questions and present information clearly and persuasively

11.10 Summary

This chapter discusses the importance of effective presentation and communication skills for healthcare professionals. It emphasizes three steps: preparation, performance, and reflection. Key strategies include managing anxiety, creating strong openings, tailoring content, simplifying content, and using storytelling. This chapter also discusses communication's role in healthcare, techniques like active listening, summarizing, and asking open-ended questions. It emphasizes overcoming barriers like time constraints and language differences. By continually refining these skills, healthcare professionals can improve patient outcomes and professional growth.

References

Calmer You. How to improve presentation skills: 10 steps to own the room. Calmer You. 2024. https://www.calmer-you.com/improve-presentation-skills/. Accessed 18 May 2004.

Duarte N. Five presentation mistakes everyone makes. Harvard Business Review. 2020. https://hbr.org/2012/12/avoid-these-five-mistakes-in-y. Accessed 30 Apr 2020.

Fatimayin F. What is communication. Lagos: National Open University of Nigeria; 2018.

Gostin I. Eight tips for delivering a great presentation. Forbes. 2022. https://www.forbes.com/sites/forbescommunicationscouncil/2022/06/14/eight-tips-for-delivering-a-great-presentation/. Accessed 16 June 2022.

Jureddi DN, Brahmaiah N. Barriers to effective communication. J Engl Lang Lit. 2016;3:114–5.

Kapur R. Barriers to effective communication. Delhi: Delhi University; 2018.

Oliveira J. Effective Communication in Healthcare Settings: Building Trust and Improving Patient Outcomes. 2024. https://doi.org/10.5281/zenodo.10946653.

Rolleter B. Presentation skills: 16 tips for effective presentations. CBS International Business School. 2024. https://www.cbs.de/en/blog/15-effective-presentation-tips-to-improve-presentation-skills/. Accessed 22 Mar 2024.

Study Skills and Lifestyle Habits That Are Conducive to Success in Education in the Health Professions

12

Khalid A. Bin Abdulrahman and Ayesha Nuzhat

Learning Objectives

1. *Master effective study techniques.*
   Develop structured study routines, utilize the SQ3R method, and apply active learning strategies to enhance academic performance in healthcare education.
2. *Adopt healthy lifestyle habits.*
   Understand the importance of balanced nutrition, quality sleep, regular exercise, and stress management in supporting academic success and overall well-being.
3. *Balance commitments and manage stress.*
   Learn strategies to harmonize academic responsibilities with social engagements, and apply mindfulness techniques to mitigate stress and prevent burnout.

12.1 Introduction

Education in the health professions requires more than merely academic skill; namely, strategic study skills and a balanced lifestyle are also necessary to overcome the difficulties presented by curricula in this context. This chapter discusses essential study tips that are important to students in the health professions. It also adopts a more in-depth approach to survey, question, read, recite, and review (SQ3R)-related methods, which are effective

K. A. Bin Abdulrahman (✉)
Department of Medical Education, College of Medicine, Imam Mohammad Ibn Saud Islamic University (IMSIU), Riyadh, Saudi Arabia
e-mail: kab@imamu.edu.sa

A. Nuzhat
Department of Anatomy and Medical Education, College of Medicine, Imam Mohammad Ibn Saud Islamic University (IMSIU), Riyadh, Saudi Arabia
e-mail: anuzhat@imamu.edu.sa

K. A. Bin Abdulrahman, H. Darami (eds.), *Essential Learning Skills for Health Professions Students*, https://doi.org/10.1007/978-981-96-5670-7_12

ways in which students can study, learn, understand, and remember important and complex information. Furthermore, it discusses mnemonics, including acronyms and pictures that can promote memory. Other significant factors in this context include health issues, such as a proper diet, healthy sleep, exercise, extracurricular activities, a balanced social life and schoolwork, avoidance of unhealthy habits, and stress management. Since students adopt healthier lifestyles as they develop their study skills, their academic performance can be enhanced, and they can become better equipped to overcome various challenges related to their healthcare professions.

A recent study highlights the significant correlation between effective study habits and academic accomplishments among medical students in Saudi Arabia (Bin Abdulrahman et al. 2021a). Key habits include time management, minimizing interruptions, goal setting, studying 3–4 hours daily, solo study for retention, using diverse learning resources, peer teaching, and strategic use of teaching materials. Motivation stems from self-gratification and family aspirations, offering valuable insights to inspire academic success and improve less accomplished students' strategies (see Table 12.1).

Table 12.1 Summary of the study habits of highly effective medical students

Category	Details
Study type	Cross-sectional observational study
Study period	September to December 2019
Participants	675 medical students (both genders) from 6 medical colleges in Saudi Arabia
Focus areas	Learning habits, prioritization, knowledge retention strategies, motivation, study hours, teaching resources
Key findings	Significant correlation between study habits and academic accomplishments
Top 10 study habits	1. Time management
	2. Avoiding interruptions (e.g. phone, family, friends)
	3. Goal setting
	4. Daily study hours: 3–4 hours
	5. Solo study for knowledge retention
	6. Using multiple learning sources
	7. Investing in technology efficiently
	8. Peer teaching
	9. Studying main lecture slides and notes (when no exams)
	10. Researching slides, notes, and previous exam questions (for exams)
Motivation factors	Self-gratification and fulfilment of family aspirations
Conclusion	Identifies effective study practices that inspire academic success and highlights strategies for improvement in less accomplished students

12.2 Tips for Effective Study Skills in the Context of Healthcare Education

12.2.1 Set a Study Time

A structured study schedule is key to the development of consistency and effective study habits in the context of healthcare education. A helpful study routine aims to provide a much-needed feeling of structure and discipline that can help address several courses involved in health profession programmes, which are often demanding (Simplilearn 2023). Setting aside a particular time for study every day can establish a routine to which students can become accustomed.

For example, a time limit during the day, such as between 7 and 9 PM, can be devoted specifically to the task of studying, thus enabling learners to stay on track with their studies. Such discipline can prepare the brain to establish a study pattern that can enable students to concentrate and absorb information easily during this time. This approach may lead to more effective and productive study sessions as the mind and body adapt to these focused learning periods.

12.2.2 Establish a Dedicated Space for Studies

A quiet, well-organized, and distraction-free environment can significantly enhance individuals' ability to concentrate and retain information. A quiet room containing an uncluttered desk, for example, can facilitate focus and thus promote substantial progress. Accordingly, students can prevent themselves from becoming distracted easily due to visual clutter since their space is well arranged and does not contain irrelevant materials. Students can also ensure that their study spaces are well illuminated and that all the materials, including textbooks and computers, are easily accessible (Hendrix 2019). Students can reserve such an area as a haven of study, thus facilitating deep thoughts and good academic performance in the context of healthcare. If students have access to such a study area, their brains always associate this place with work, thus separating time spent in such an area from students' free time or relaxation time.

12.2.3 Use the Study Sandwich Technique

The *study sandwich* technique involves strategically organizing study sessions to maximize focus and efficiency. Here is how it works:

1. *Difficult Subject in the Middle*: Place the challenging or demanding subject matter between two easier topics. This approach ensures that the most strenuous part of studying is surrounded by less taxing material, helping to maintain momentum and motivation.
2. *Stay on Schedule*: Avoid falling behind. If you do, use the weekend to catch up and get back on track.
3. *Prioritize Current Material*: Focus on the most recent topics or material first to stay aligned with current lectures or courses.
4. *Value Your Time*: Avoid wasting time, as it significantly impacts your chances of success.

This method is designed to improve productivity and maintain a balanced study routine, combining focus on difficult areas with time management strategies (Bin Abdulrahman et al. 2021b) (Fig. 12.1).

12.2.4 Break Study Time into Sessions

Short, focused study sessions can improve students' focus and information retention, even with regard to highly intensive subjects such as healthcare education. For example, the

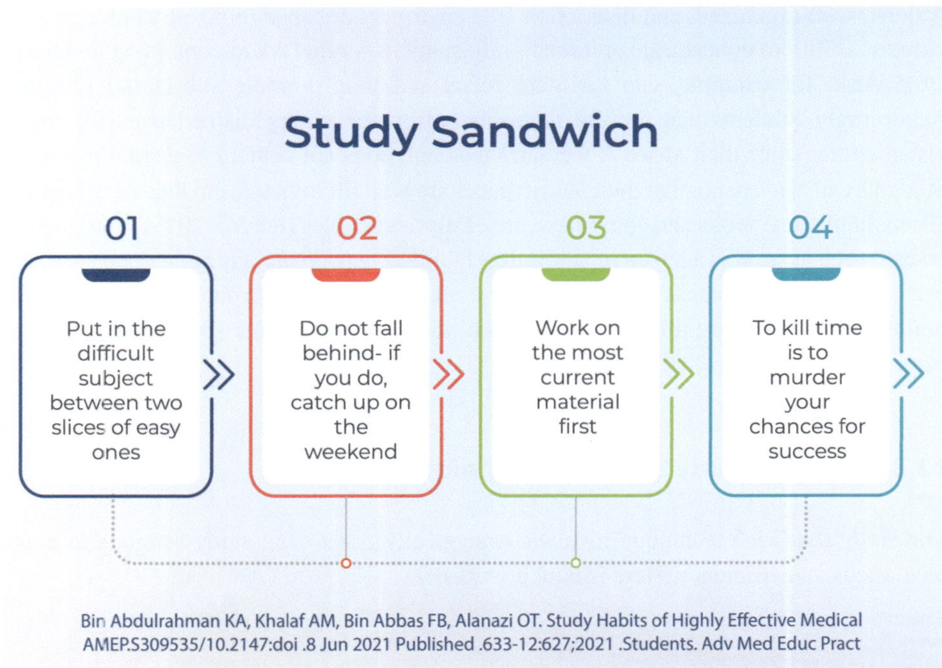

Fig.12.1 A visual representation of the study sandwich technique

Pomodoro technique involves dividing one's study time into digestible sections of 25–30 minutes each, which are followed by short breaks. This approach helps students avoid mental fatigue, maintain high levels of productivity, and study more easily. Accordingly, short periods of concentrated study work perfectly alongside the natural attention span of the brain. When students work in such bursts, they are highly focused and can thus grasp information more effectively (TutorLyft 2024). Regular breaks offer the mind time to relax and refocus on what the material that must be grasped—this approach thus prevents burnout and enhances students' motivation throughout the studying process. It allows students to stand up, stretch, retrieve healthy snacks, or even go for a short walk. After the fourth iteration of this pattern, a longer pause (i.e. 15 minutes or longer) enables students to rest more effectively. Such cycles conserve students' focus and energy, thus making their work more viable and allowing it nearly to resemble child's play.

12.2.5 Study Actively

Active study techniques are critical in health education since they can deepen students' ability to understand and retain information. In contrast to passive reading or listening, active studying involves asking questions, discussing, and applying the knowledge that one has obtained (Broadbent 2021). This approach allows for interaction with the subject; thus, learning becomes more dynamic. For example, self-quizzing is a compelling active study approach that allows students to challenge themselves to repeat essential concepts and questions. This approach allows students to help highlight areas of a paper that require further review if they are to retain the corresponding knowledge. Another powerful method used in learning is group discussion, which involves explicating concepts among group members, debating different viewpoints, and solving problems. This approach enhances students' understanding and helps them acquire important practical skills pertaining to communication and teamwork that are key in healthcare settings.

12.2.6 Take Notes in Class

Note-taking is a significant facilitator of memory and learning in the context of healthcare. The activity involved in note-taking is effective if a student can note the main points of the given material actively, thus producing a resource document pertaining to the event in question that may subsequently be reviewed. According to Courtie (2022), another effective note-taking strategy is the Cornell method, which requires students to divide the page on which notes are written into three sections: a narrow left-hand column that contains keywords or questions, a wider right-hand column that supports detailed note-taking, and a section for summary at the bottom of the page. Students can list key ideas and details presented in the main lecture in the right-hand column, while on the left side, they write questions or keywords that can support their memory after class (Nachiappan 2022). For

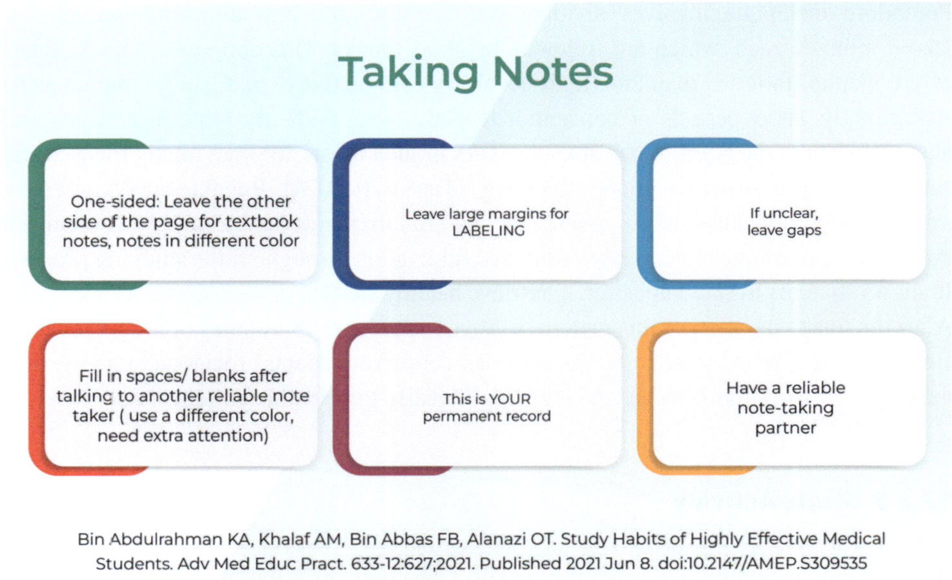

Fig. 12.2 Illustration of a systematic note-taking approach

example, as illustrated below, in a lecture on cardiovascular physiology, students may write detailed notes regarding the operations of the heart in the right-hand column, while the left-hand column could include key terms (Fig. 12.2).

12.2.7 Summarize or Teach What One Has Learned

Summarizing materials or explaining them to somebody else can increase students' comprehension and retention in extraordinary cases. Such active learning activities force students to process and reframe information in their own words, thus allowing them to relearn the material and increasing their actual understanding thereof.

Another powerful technique that can support the further absorption of learning involves teaching the material in question to someone else. This strategy is known as the Feynman technique, and it involves explaining a concept in simple terms or in a straightforward and elementary way (Cam 2023). To describe anything adequately, one must thoroughly understand the material in question step by step until it has been completed updated in one's mind. This approach enables students to clarify the issue at hand and reveals areas that they have not yet fully understood. For example, study groups, during which students take turns teaching each other, can be very helpful. Each student may summarize some portion of the relevant material and then explain it to others. Since the process of reviewing this material is shared, this methodology usually fosters participation, helps students develop communication skills, and allows different students to highlight different dimensions of the same material.

12.3 Use the SQ3R Method

12.3.1 Survey

Surveying the material at hand represents the first step in the SQ3R method; this approach helps the student become familiar with the material before beginning the process of intense reading. Students scan the text in question quickly to determine its structure, thereby developing a preconceived mental framework for the information that they will learn at this level (Nebel 2022). During the scanning process, students must identify all the features that stand out to them, such as headings, subheadings, graphs, charts, items printed in bold, and any text that is printed in a different colour or font. Your sentence is clear but can be slightly refined for improved flow and precision. Here's a polished version:
These indicate and provide clues not only about the main topics addressed in the material, but also about the organization of the content. By employing this strategy, students can improve their study practices, understand complex information, and recall the material in question, thus preparing them to interact with the material during the study and allowing them to obtain an overview of the text.

12.3.2 Question

The Q in SQ3R refers to the process of asking questions with regard to the surveyed material. In this step, students' relatively passive reading is transformed into an active learning process, in which learners engage critically with the text on the basis of an established purpose regarding the information that they seek to understand (Nebel 2022). Proposing relevant questions entails that students' reading has a purpose and offers them the opportunity to focus on the material, thus supporting their understanding. By employing this method, a reader can pose specific questions during the reading process and concentrate on finding answers to those questions.

For example, after the students read a chapter titled 'Cardiac Cycle,' they may generate related questions, such as the following:

'How is the heart rate regulated?'

Writing these questions down before reading helps the student remain highly focused. Thus, reading involves answering these questions, thereby reinforcing the reader's understanding and retention of similar information. This approach can thus enhance students' understanding and prepare them for examinations and practical application in the healthcare programme.

12.3.3 Read

The third step involved in the SQ3R method entails reading with relevant questions in mind prepared during the previewing process. Accordingly, the reader can be challenged to read with a continual sense of purpose and to answer these questions, thereby acquiring a deep understanding of the content (Nebel 2022). While reading, students should attempt to answer the corresponding questions.

For example, a student must answer the following question: 'What are the different stages of the cardiac cycle?' The student must thus review the stages of the cardiac cycle and identify the various stages alongside their characteristics. As students read, they should highlight or underline key points, make annotations in the margins, and summarize important concepts in their own words. Reading the material with the goals of answering direct questions and producing concise notes further increases students' ability to understand and remember what they read.

12.3.4 Recite

Step four in the SQ3R method involves reciting the material in an individual's own words. This step represents an active learning technique that can promote comprehension and retention by encouraging information processing and articulation in the learner's own words. Reciting involves summarizing parts of the material aloud or explaining important points either to oneself or others. This approach helps students not only to consolidate what they have learned but also to clarify areas of confusion (Nebel 2022). For example, after reading a paragraph concerning the phases of the cardiac cycle, the student might summarize the information, indicate what each phase does in a summary, and then comment on the relevance of each phase in his or her own words. Students can also discuss heart rate regulation systems or variables that affect cardiac output. In healthcare education, it is crucial to understand the subject matter to ensure that one is prepared for both tests and real-world applications.

12.3.5 Review

The final step in the SQ3R method involves reviewing the material by answering the formulated questions once again, this time without referring to any notes. This step tests students' comprehension and retention of the material. Performing such an exercise after study would be useful, as it can help identify areas that require further study. This review process allows students to reinforce learning and ensure that they have obtained an embedded understanding of critical concepts (Nebel 2022). For example, a student may ask a question such as 'What are the different phases of the cardiac cycle?' The student would then be expected to recall and describe each of these phases without consulting their notes.

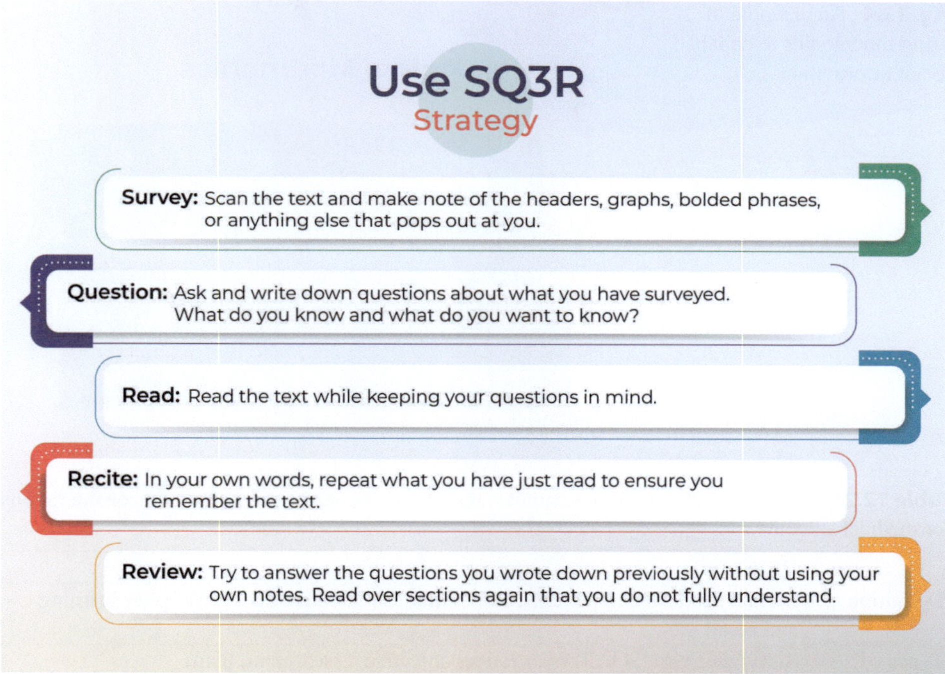

Fig. 12.3 The SQ3R strategy: a systematic approach for improving reading capacity

This technique is essential with respect to students' long-term retention of material and their success in terms of both examinations and practical applications throughout the process of healthcare education. Figure 12.3 summarizes the SQ3R method.

12.4 Use Mnemonics

The term 'mnemonics' refers to the devices that are used to remember information by connecting new concepts with existing structures of memory. Mnemonic devices include acronyms, image associations, and coined sayings (Fig. 12.4).

12.4.1 Acronyms

Acronyms are words or phrases that are created on the basis of the initials of or occasionally several letters from string of words; these letters then represent the information or concepts to be retained (Table 12.2). For example, RICE is a commonly used acronym for rest, ice, compression, and elevation. This acronym is commonly used in the process of treating typical injuries, including sprains and strains. Each letter of the acronym represents a particular step in this process:

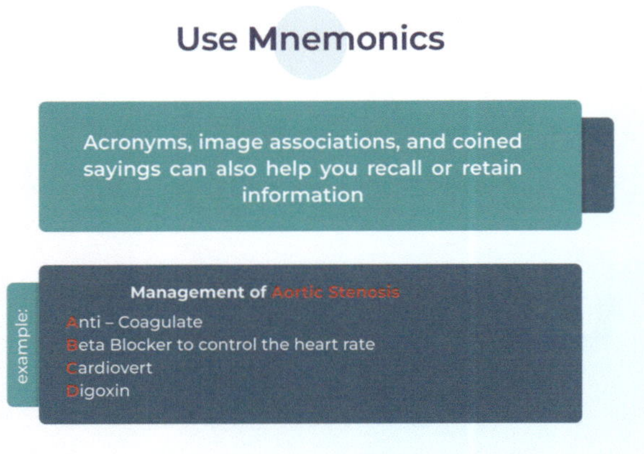

Fig. 12.4 An example of using mnemonics to enhance recall information

Table 12.2 A concise overview of mnemonics, their types, benefits, examples, and considerations for medical students

	Details
Definition	Memory tools using patterns, associations, or creative cues to simplify learning and recall
Types	*Acronyms*: e.g. 'SOAP' (subjective, objective, assessment, plan)
	Rhymes/Phrases: e.g. 'Some Lovers Try Positions…' for carpal bones
	Chunking: Breaking info into smaller parts
	Visualization: Linking info to vivid mental images
	Stories/Analogies: Relating concepts to narratives
Advantages	*Retention*: Memorize complex details easily
	Recall: Retrieve info quickly during exams or practice
	Engagement: Makes learning interactive and enjoyable
Examples	*Cranial nerves*: 'Oh, Oh, Oh, To Touch And Feel Very Good Velvet, Such Heaven'
	Clinical signs: 'BEARS' (bloating, emesis, anorexia, rebound tenderness, shifting pain)
	Pharmacology: 'ABCDEF' for corticosteroid side effects
Best practices	Personalize mnemonics for better memory
	Combine with understanding for deeper learning
	Repeat often to reinforce memory
Limitations	Overdependence may hinder conceptual understanding
	Complex mnemonics can be hard to remember without context

Rest: Refrain from using the injured area.

Ice: Use ice to ease swelling.

Compression: Compress the part in question using a bandage with the aim of preventing swelling.

Elevation: Raise the injured area above the level of the heart to minimize swelling.

12.4.2 Image Associations

Image association is a method in which concepts are remembered on the basis of pictorial imagery. For example, the brain may be more likely to recognize a photo more than a corresponding description, and image association may thus lead to significant improvements in memory (Radović and Manzey 2019). For example, a student can use mental images of the heart's structure to facilitate information retrieval.

12.4.3 Coined Sayings

Mnemonics can also use coined sayings, which refer to short, easy-to-remember phrases or sentences that provide necessary information. Coined sayings often use rhyme to enhance the process of memorization. The sequence of mitosis includes interphase, monophase, metaphase, anaphase, and telophase. Many coined sayings have been developed to help people remember these phases, for example, 'I Paint My Aunt's Toy.'

In short, try to master the art of smart studying with effective strategies, namely structured study breaks, summarization, self-assessment, mnemonics, and the SQ3R method, all tailored for a positive and engaging learning experience (Fig. 12.5).

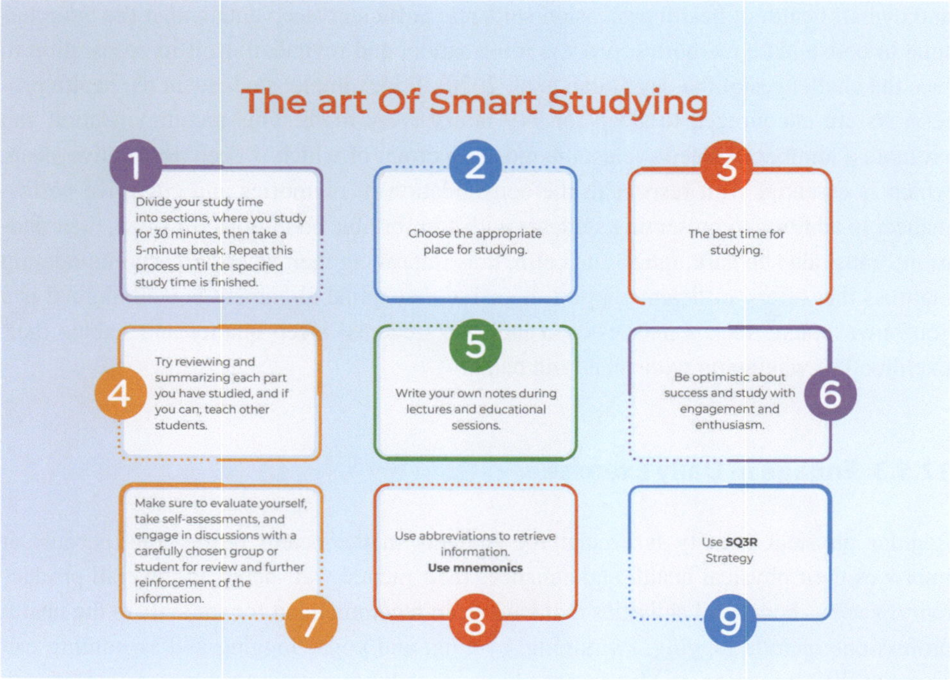

Fig. 12.5 Master the art of smart studying with effective strategies

12.5 Good Lifestyle Habits for Effective Students in the Health Professions

12.5.1 Eat a Healthy Diet

Eating a healthy diet is a critical element for students in the health professions because it promotes energy, mental clarity, and general health. Good nutrition allows the brain to obtain all the nutrients that it needs to ensure effective functioning; in turn, nutrients that enhance thinking ability, alertness, and memory are critical ingredients that can promote excellence in the intense curriculum for all healthcare providers (Cena and Calder 2020). A balanced diet should consist of many nutrient-dense foods, including fruits, vegetables, lean proteins, and whole grains, as illustrated in Fig. 12.2. For example, students can begin with entire grains and proteins, such as oats with nuts and fruit or scrambled eggs with whole-grain toast and avocado. Awareness of good choices in nutrition is associated with better grades in school and can help lay a solid foundation for future efforts to promote health and wellness.

12.5.2 Maintain Quality Sleep

Adequate quality sleep is crucial with respect to the cognitive processes, emotional health, and overall health of health profession students. Sufficient sleep entails that the brain has time to consolidate memories, process information, and revitalize itself in preparation to face the challenges of the day (Jalali et al. 2020). For example, students in the health professions are encouraged to sleep for 7–9 hours every night. This recommendation can promote a number of sleep cycles, the most important of which is deep, restorative sleep, which is essential with respect to the consolidation of memories and cognitive performance. In addition to presenting students with comfortable conditions for sleep, their bedrooms must also be dark, quiet, and calm, thus improving their sleep. An accommodating mattress that offers sufficient support to ensure that spinal alignment is well aligned is a good investment; such a mattress can increase students' sleep quality and reduce their likelihood of waking up with aches and pains.

12.5.3 Engage in Daily Exercise

Regular physical activity is crucial for students in the health professions because it improves their physical health and enhances their mental well-being and overall productivity. Various beneficial activities that have been recommended for students in the health professions include jogging, swimming, cycling, and yoga. Jogging and swimming can promote the circulation of blood to the brain, thereby facilitating the generation of new brain cells and increasing cognitive capacity (Rodríguez-Romo et al. 2022). For example, students majoring in the health professions can incorporate exercise into their daily routines, such as by taking regular walks to break up their study hours, attending group exercise classes at recreation centres, or learning yoga with the goals of promoting relaxation and stress management. Owing to the intensive nature of their education, regular exercise is essential for stress management among these students.

12.5.4 Engage in Extracurricular Activities

Extracurricular activities play a significant role in the growth of health professionals. Some such activities greatly enhance individuals' most basic yet critical skills that can be attained outside the classroom; namely, interactions with other people in this context can allow such students to feel balanced and fulfilled. A good example of this benefit pertaining to students in the health professions focuses on clubs pertaining to this career path, such as medical or nursing student associations (Chen et al. 2023). Most of these clubs offer networking opportunities, resources, and discussions regarding various topics or issues pertaining to individuals' studies. Students can thus excel academically by participation in extracurricular activities; thus, such activities are not only permissible but also help prepare the student for life, academic excellence, and all-rounded existence, thus allowing them to face the numerous challenges and responsibilities that lie ahead in their careers in healthcare.

12.5.5 Establish a Balance Between Social and Academic Commitments

Students in the health professions can balance their social commitments with their academic commitments with the goals of preventing burnout and maintaining their well-being. Students should seek to establish an equitable equilibrium among meaningful and engaging social relationships, class work, and well-being. One strategy that can be used to prioritize one's activities in descending order of importance involves identifying and merging the most critical academic duties, which can be addressed first (Chen et al. 2023). Additionally, a priority matrix that arranges tasks according to urgency and importance ensures that high-priority tasks are performed before less critical tasks.

Setting realistic goals is another relevant factor in this context. Dividing significant projects and assignments into small portions that can be completed before specific deadlines helps students avoid overwhelming feelings and makes it easy for them to advance step by step (Chen et al. 2023). This approach enables a person to stay focused on a given time without becoming mentally tired, particularly on the basis of the Pomodoro technique, which is a particular work-break formula that is divided into blocks consisting of 25 minutes each. Accordingly, students can manage to maintain their social and academic status.

12.5.6 Avoid Smoking and Unhealthy Habits

Smoking is a behaviour that represents one of the most significant health threats, and students in the health professions are no exception to the need to manage their performance and promote their health in this regard. This behaviour is associated with several risks, including respiratory and cardiovascular diseases (Hjort et al. 2022). Such health problems might damage the student's attentiveness, decrease their stamina, and, as a result, lead to high levels of absenteeism that can lead the student astray from the right path in terms of educational experience and success.

Unhealthy habits, such as consuming excessive amounts of alcohol, eating inappropriate foods, and sustained inactivity, may lead to poor health, thereby weakening students. Such habits may be the cause of chronic conditions such as obesity, diabetes, and mental disorders, which further undermine students' health and quality of life (Hjort et al. 2022). When students avoid smoking and other risky activities, we observe significant improvements in their physical health, mental well-being, and academic performance.

12.5.7 Implement Stress Management Techniques

Effective stress management is mandatory for students in the health professions as a result of the pressure associated with the academic and clinical requirements that they face. Namely, effective strategies against chronic stress should be employed, as they may lead to the emergence of various mental and physical disorders, including burnout, anxiety, depression, and decreased academic performance (Chen et al. 2023). One of the most frequently recommended techniques for stress management is mindfulness. In general, remaining present and deepening one's engagement with the current moment enables them to reduce stress and improve their concentration. Students can easily be taught practices in this manner, which can then be incorporated into their daily routines; for instance, in the context of mindful breathing, students seek to focus on their breath.

12.6 Summary and Conclusion

This chapter discussed the central aspects of practical study skills and healthy living in the context of students in the health professions. It began by emphasizing that students should establish a set study time and dedicated space for study and break their study time into manageable sessions, followed by active study techniques such as note-making and teaching others the material they seek to learn. The application of the SQ3R method, including the strategies of survey, question, read, recite, and review, as well as the use of mnemonics to increase retention were also discussed.

Additionally, this chapter discussed the reasons underlying these good lifestyle practices. We recommended a diet that focuses on fruits, vegetables, lean proteins, and whole

Table 12.3 Summary of the lifestyle habits of highly effective medical students

Aspect	Details
Study type	Multi-institutional, cross-sectional observational study conducted in six medical colleges in Saudi Arabia
Study period	September to December 2019
Participants	675 medical students (50% male), aged 18–24
Sleep	87.6% slept 4–8 hours daily; 44% dissatisfied with sleep
Eating habits	28.1% had three meals daily; ~40% skipped breakfast; 44% ate fast food regularly
Water intake	44.7% drank 2 L of water daily
Coffee consumption	63.3% drank black coffee daily; females consumed more coffee than males ($p < 0.001$)
Physical activity	Only 4.3% exercised for 30+ minutes daily
Social life	65% were introverted; 81% were somewhat satisfied or satisfied with social life; males were more satisfied than females ($p = 0.001$)
Smoking habits	4.6% smoked cigarettes daily; 7.1% used e-cigarettes daily (more males, $p < 0.001$); 0.3% used shisha daily
Leisure activities	Top 5: Social media (75.9%), movies (61.3%), friends (58.1%), family (55.4%), Internet (53.6%)
Gender differences	Males consumed more fast food and e-cigarettes Females preferred social media and movies
Conclusion	Healthy lifestyles to some extent, with notable sex-based differences in physical activity and eating habits

grains as the best sources of proper, balanced nutrition. This research highlights the importance of sleep and posits that 7–9 hours at night are required for quality sleep, thus improving our cognition and health. We reiterated the benefits of regular exercise and recommended activities such as jogging, swimming, and yoga; we also highlighted the importance of engaging in extracurricular activities that can promote personal growth. Moreover, one must learn how to balance social demands with academic demands to curb burnout and to prevent smoking and other unhealthy behaviours. This finding once again highlights the need to continue stress management techniques, including mindfulness, meditation, and counselling. These practices should help ensure that students are well prepared to overcome the high-stress demands pertaining to competence and resilience in the profession that are associated with healthcare careers (Table 12.3).

References

Bin Abdulrahman KA, Khalaf AM, Bin Abbas FB, Alanazi OT. Study habits of highly effective medical students. Adv Med Educ Pract. 2021a;12:627–33. https://doi.org/10.2147/AMEP.S309535. PMID: 34135654; PMCID: PMC8197661.

Bin Abdulrahman KA, Khalaf AM, Bin Abbas FB, Alanezi OT. The lifestyle of Saudi medical students. Int J Environ Res Public Health. 2021b;18(15):7869. https://doi.org/10.3390/ijerph18157869. PMID: 34360161; PMCID: PMC8345573.

Broadbent K. 6 active study techniques that actually work. Online courses and university preparation from expert tutors. 2021. https://www.melioeducation.com/blog/active-study-techniques-that-actually-work/.

Cam. The Feynman technique. A&S Academic Advising and Coaching. 2023. https://www.colorado.edu/artssciences-advising/resource-library/life-skills/the-feynman-technique-in-academic-coaching.

Cena H, Calder PC. Defining a healthy diet: evidence for the role of contemporary dietary patterns in health and disease. Nutrients. 2020;12:334.

Chen C, Bian F, Zhu Y. The relationship between social support and academic engagement among university students: the chain mediating effects of life satisfaction and academic motivation. BMC Public Health. 2023;23:2368–8.

Courtie B. Seven effective note taking strategies for university students. Online courses and university preparation from expert tutors. 2022. https://www.melioeducation.com/blog/note-taking-strategies-for-university-students/.

Hendrix E. How your surroundings affect the way you study. UCAS. 2019. https://www.ucas.com/connect/blogs/how-your-surroundings-affect-way-you-study.

Hjort AV, Kuipers MAG, Stage M, Pisinger C, Klinker CD. Intervention activities associated with the implementation of a comprehensive school tobacco policy at Danish vocational schools: a repeated cross-sectional study. Int J Environ Res Public Health. 2022;19:12489.

Jalali R, Khazaei H, Paveh BK, Hayrani Z, Menati L. The effect of sleep quality on students' academic achievement. Adv Med Educ Pract. 2020;11:497–502.

Nachiappan S. Note-taking and note-making: the ever-cherished art! Indian J Ophthalmol. 2022;70:4438–44.

Nebel C. SQ3R or read, recite, review. The Learning Scientists. 2022. https://www.learningscientists.org/blog/2021/3/4-1.

Radović T, Manzey D. The impact of a mnemonic acronym on learning and performing a procedural task and its resilience toward interruptions. Front Psychol. 2019;10:2522.

Rodríguez-Romo G, Acebes-Sánchez J, García-Merino S, Garrido-Muñoz M, Blanco-García C, Diez-Vega I. Physical activity and mental health in undergraduate students. Int J Environ Res Public Health. 2022;20:195.

Simplilearn. 10 time management skills and techniques for students. Simplilearn.com. 2023. https://www.simplilearn.com/tutorials/time-management-tutorial/best-time-management-tips-for-students.

TutorLyft. The dos and don'ts of study breaks: maximizing productivity and rest. 2024. https://www.tutorlyft.com/blogs/the-dos-and-donts-of-study-breaks.

Concept Mapping for Students in Health Professions: Enhancing Education and Application

13

Khalid A. Bin Abdulrahman and Salah-Ud-Din Khan

Learning Objectives

1. *Understand the structure and components of concept maps.*
   Learners will be able to identify the key elements of concept maps, including nodes and linking lines, and differentiate between hierarchical and nonhierarchical structures.
2. *Apply concept mapping techniques in healthcare education.*
   Learners will demonstrate the ability to use concept maps for organizing, synthesizing, and visualizing complex healthcare topics to enhance learning, identify knowledge gaps, and foster critical thinking.
3. *Develop collaborative and critical thinking skills.*
   Learners will engage in collaborative concept mapping activities to improve teamwork, communication, and interdisciplinary collaboration, while fostering problem-solving and reflective practices in healthcare contexts.

K. A. Bin Abdulrahman (✉)
Department of Medical Education, College of Medicine, Imam Mohammad Ibn Saud Islamic University (IMSIU), Riyadh, Saudi Arabia
e-mail: kab@imamu.edu.sa

S. Khan
Department of Biochemistry, College of Medicine, Imam Mohammad Ibn Saud Islamic University (IMSIU), Riyadh, Saudi Arabia
e-mail: sdikhan@imamu.edu.sa

K. A. Bin Abdulrahman, H. Darami (eds.), *Essential Learning Skills for Health Professions Students*, https://doi.org/10.1007/978-981-96-5670-7_13

13.1 Introduction

Concept maps are graphic tools for depicting knowledge and concepts to help visualize and structure information. The objective of this chapter is to clearly describe the structure and components of a concept map; its practical application within education for healthcare professionals; and specific examples in medicine, nursing, and applied health sciences. This chapter analyzes these aspects to emphasize the importance of concept mapping in providing a more profound understanding, enhancing assessment techniques, and stimulating cooperative learning among future healthcare professionals.

13.2 Understanding Concept Maps, Structures, and Components

13.2.1 Concept Maps

Concept maps are graphical tools for organizing and representing knowledge. They visually represent the relationships between concepts, ideas, or information in a hierarchical format. A specific topic is at the center of a concept map surrounded by related ideas or subtopics (Interaction Design Foundation 2016). Various concept maps exist, including spider maps, flowcharts used to depict processes, hierarchy maps used to visualize organizations, and system maps used to visualize systems. These concepts can be interconnected by labelled lines or arrows (as shown in Fig. 13.1).

Concept maps can be used for anything: brainstorming, problem-solving, planning, study, or information presentation. They allow a student to break down a complex subject into small and understandable parts, showing how they relate (Interaction Design Foundation 2016). They also promote cooperation between individuals if they are working with/investigating the same project or ordinary subject matter. These concept maps enable users to present their thoughts coherently in a structure and, therefore, help in understanding an issue while also making it possible to pinpoint any gaps in knowledge. These flexible tools can be used in ways that suit individual learners and their preferences, thus providing them with resources for education research and professional practice. Figure 13.2 shows a hierarchical concept map—for example, one illustrating the nursing care of diabetes.

13.2.2 Structure

Two essential elements organize a concept map: nodes and linking lines. Nodes are considered the basic units of concept maps; in other words, they represent single concepts, ideas, or elements related to the subject (Ligita et al. 2020). Those concepts may vary from

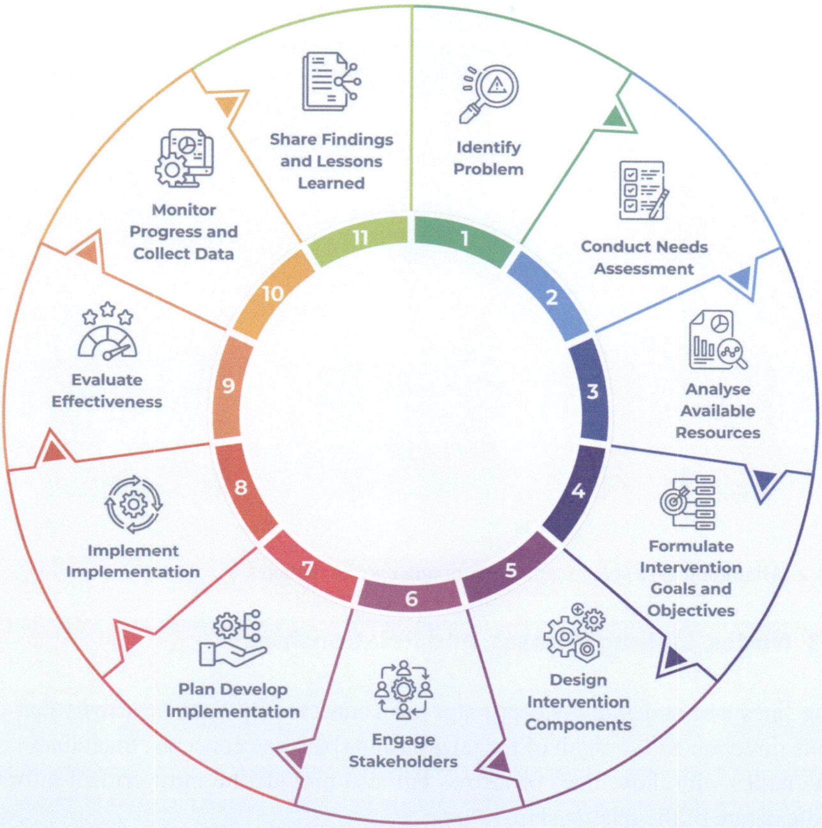

Fig. 13.1 Flowchart concept map for obesity intervention

general terms to abstract ideas, theories, or principles. As a rule, a single node is consistently visible within the map, which makes it easy to recognize and distinguish. Each node serves as a visual container: one thing holding a particular notion in place and one of the centers on a map.

Linking lines, also known as connecting lines or arrows, allow for relationships between nodes; they indicate the links or associations among the ideas represented by the nodes. These linking lines are labels or descriptors added along the lines joining the corresponding nodes (Ligita et al. 2020). They specify the nature of the link, whether it is causal in character, a relationship, an order of occurrence, or another type of link.

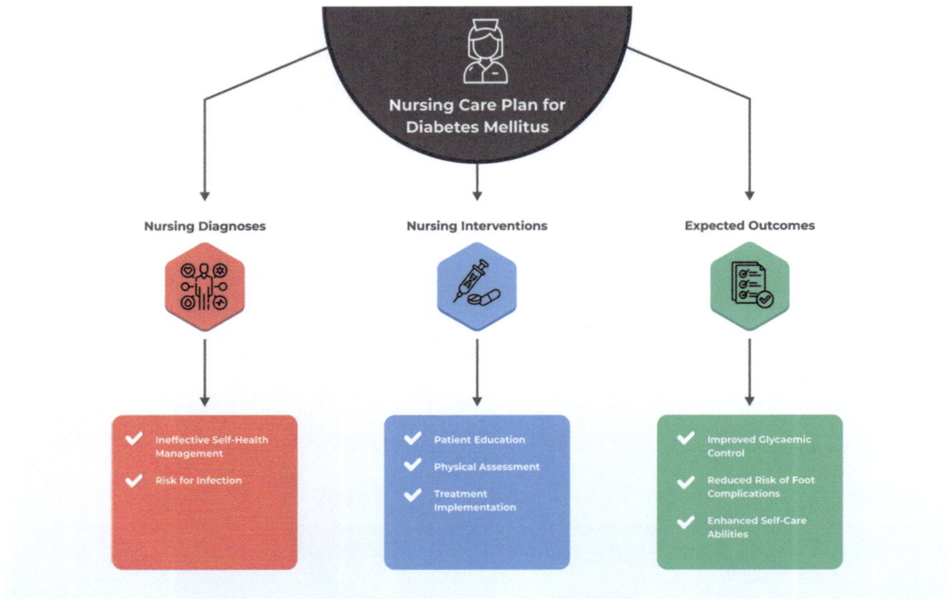

Fig. 13.2 Hierarchical concept map, e.g., nursing care of diabetes

13.2.3 Nodes, Linking Phrases, and Relationships

Linking lines and nodes in concept maps are connected by lines or arrows that clearly show the direction and strength of the relationships between concepts. Such lines not only link the nodes with those lines or arrows but also provide the most critical information about the nature of the relationship.

The relationships between nodes, either through lines or arrows, are indicated by linking phrases that show the directionality of those relationships. Arrows generally describe the relationship between two terms as "causes" or "leads to," showing the direction of the relationship or sequence of events from one concept to another (Ligita et al. 2020). On the other hand, lines without arrows describe nondirectional relationships, such as "is related to" or "is associated with," expressing mutuality of being, whereby the concepts refer to each other without designating the nature of the reference.

In a concept map, the lines or arrows also depict the relative strength or importance of the interconcept relationships. The width, length, and curvature of the lines could indicate varying relationships. Thicker lines or smaller distances between nodes generally indicate stronger relationships where the importance or relevance of the connection is given (Ligita et al. 2020). In contrast, weaker or less prevalent relationships between the concepts in the map are suggested by thinner lines or longer distances.

13.2.4 Hierarchical and Nonhierarchical Structures

Concept maps are flexible in their organization; they can be hierarchical or nonhierarchical depending on the developer's preference and the topic under consideration. In hierarchical maps, more general concepts are commonly depicted above more profound, specific concepts. This tree structure has a central point on which the main ideas are written, which extends to larger subconcepts that look like branches and, finally, to even more minor details, similar to leaves (Baliga et al. 2021). They provide an excellent graphic representation of the systematic relationships among knowledge parts, emphasizing the links between topics and their respective subtopics.

On the other hand, nonhierarchical concept maps do not have such strictly top-down arrangements and appear more dispersed and interconnected. In other words, this type of map organizes concepts based on thematic or conceptual similarities rather than placing them in hierarchical order (Baliga et al. 2021). Concepts are often related on several levels, implying a broader vision of the relationships among different ideas. This flexible, nonhierarchical structure allows exploration, where individuals can make discoveries to gain a more pronounced understanding of subjects and think creatively.

13.3 Practical Applications of Concept Maps in Healthcare Education

13.3.1 Learning Tools for Students

Concept maps are helpful learning tools for most health education students because they elicit activities wherein students interact with the study material. They help organize and integrate new information (Fonseca et al. 2023). A concept map allows students to organize complicated information schematically. By creating concept maps, students can draw conceptual relationships between various concepts, theories, and components related to their studies in a visible manner. This visual nature helps learners subdivide large quantities of information into small elements that are easier to understand and remember. Moreover, concept maps similarly elicit active learning, unlike the passive activity of taking in information. When making concept maps, learners must process and synthesize information, build relationships between the concepts, and work out how these relationships relate to others. Hence, the learner is more active in learning and understands the materials more deeply. Figure 13.3 demonstrates an example of concept map for differential diagnosis.

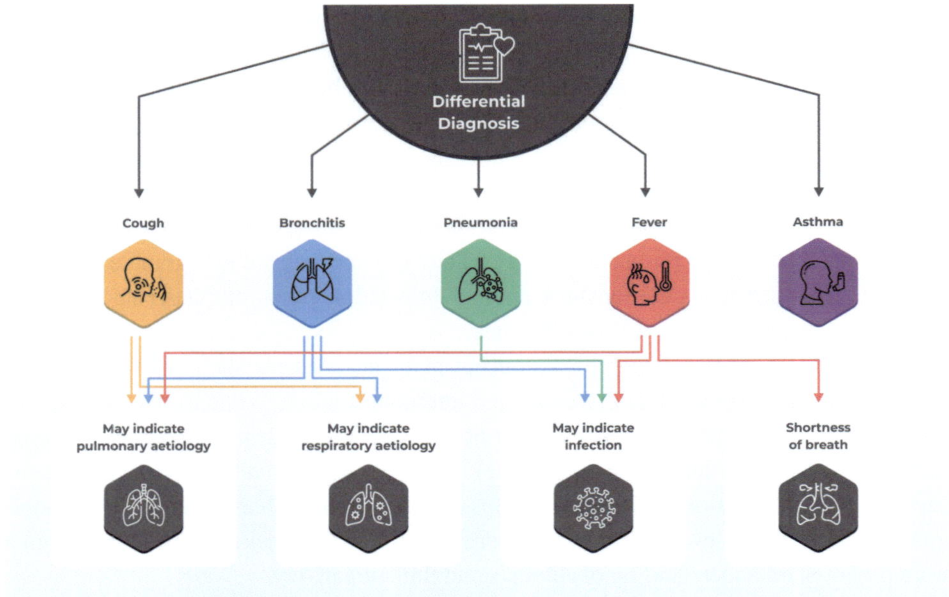

Fig. 13.3 Concept map for differential diagnosis

13.3.2 Knowledge Gaps

Concept maps help learners identify their knowledge gaps and see the connections between topics in a subject area.

Visual Representation Concept maps visually represent the relationships of the concepts to the topic. They help learners visualize the concepts and their relationships, revealing where they might lack understanding or miss connections.

Hierarchy and Structure In a hierarchical concept map, broader concepts can be located at the top with more specific concepts branching below them. With this structure in place, learners can easily see the main themes and how they relate to more detailed concepts (Joshi et al. 2022). Thus, they will easily find gaps when branches within the hierarchy are missing or some connections are absent.

Linking Phrases The linking phrases in concept maps are important because they explain how the nodes are related. Linking phrases explain how concepts relate to one another through cause–effect relationships, associations, or simple relationships (Joshi et al. 2022). By checking for these linking phrases, learners can determine what relationships exist between topics and detect where connections might be weak or absent.

Active Engagement Concept maps must be constructed as they engage the learner. By building a map, learners can think critically about how concepts relate to one another and how they can be linked (Joshi et al. 2022). Hence, not only will learners be able to identify gaps by relating different topics, but they will also draw the linkages between those topics.

Concept maps are potent instruments for identifying knowledge gaps and connecting topics associated with a subject.

13.3.3 Long-Term Retention and Deep Understanding

Concept maps also significantly enhance long-term retention and deepen the understanding of the subject matter.

Information Organization Concept maps organize information through a visual representation in a structure. Such deep involvement in the learning process allows learners to understand details by encouraging them to think critically about relationships between concepts and how those relationships relate to real-world scenarios (Nicoara et al. 2020).

Create Meaningful Learning Concept maps facilitate meaningful learning for learners trying to relate what they are learning to what they already know (Nicoara et al. 2020). When learners develop new concepts in their concept maps and link them to those learned earlier, they start to have a more coherent grasp of the topic, enhancing retention over time.

Visualizations Concept maps are highly visual tools that give form to conceptual material, rendering it somewhat tangible and easy to grasp. Since information is provided graphically, concept maps address students of different orientations and help them visualize data (Nicoara et al. 2020). They facilitate memory encoding by learners, thus allowing them to more easily remember information at a later time.

13.4 Effective Tool for Assessment and Evaluation

13.4.1 Assessing Student Knowledge

Educators can use concept maps to assess students: preassessment is the process through which teachers may require students to develop a concept map that illustrates what they know about the subject matter before embarking on a new topic (Eachempati et al. 2020). Through preassessment, teachers uncover students' prior knowledge and misconceptions, enabling them to tailor instructions to the specific learning needs of their students.

Formative Assessment Educators can use concept maps to help students understand essential concepts when learning. Learners can create individual or collaborative concept maps on paper and digitally to organize and represent educational material (Eachempati et al. 2020).

13.4.2 Evaluation of Student Understanding

The accuracy and completeness of concept maps are critical indicators of students' understanding and proficiency in a particular subject. The representation of relevant concepts and an accurate depiction indicate a grasp of the subject matter on the part of the student (Tarım et al. 2022). Accuracy in representing concepts ensures that a student is thoroughly grounded in the knowledge and central principles or ideas under the topic.

Depth of Elaboration The completeness of a concept map also indicates a student's depth of understanding of a subject. A richer concept map, with more detailed explanations, examples, and descriptions, shows that the student more deeply understands the material (Tarım et al. 2022). Those who can describe subtly and elaborate on connections between concepts are more than just students with superficial knowledge; they have developed a deeper understanding.

Identification of Knowledge Gaps Incomplete or inaccurate concept maps can also indicate areas where students' understanding can be improved. Therefore, educators who have developed their students' concept maps can identify these gaps and provide targeted support or further instruction to help students better conceptualize misconceived topics or topics in which they are weak (Tarım et al. 2022). By monitoring the accuracy and completeness of concept maps, an educator can identify areas in which further instruction is needed to improve knowledge accurately.

13.4.3 Collaborative Learning Environments

Students can develop concept maps using collaborative strategies and technologies in a cooperative learning environment. The following describes how students work with each other to create effective concept maps.

Group Brainstorming The students begin with a group brainstorming session. They discuss the main ideas of the subject and further outline a list of ideas they plan to incorporate into their concept map (Mende et al. 2020). In this case, group brainstorming helps students discover related concepts and relationships using the views and knowledge of other students.

Division of Activities When the critical concepts in the question have been identified, tasks may be divided and allocated between group members to generate the concept map. Each student in the group can participate in researching and placing specific concepts or relationships on the map (Mende et al. 2020). This division ensures that the load is fairly distributed and that each student does his or her best to develop the concept map.

Discussion and Reflection Knowledge is constructed when students generate a concept map through discussion and reflection. Such knowledge can be further expanded as students discuss how different concepts relate, debate interpretations from different standpoints, and reflect on what they have learned (Mende et al. 2020). Discussions and reflections facilitate active learning and critical thinking; hence, a quality concept map is realized.

Finalization and Presentation Once a concept map has been completed, students should run through the map with peer reviewers and refine it. The students could then present the map to the class or submit it to the instructor for grading. Presenting the concept map should allow the students to demonstrate their understanding of the subject being offered to their respective peers and instructors. Thus, collaborative learning environments are essential opportunities for students to work together in creating concept maps.

13.4.4 Benefits of Teamwork, Communication, and Idea Exchange

Working as a team, communicating, and sharing ideas are vital components of a learning environment. Thus, several advantages arise when students work together to create concept maps.

Better Learning Outcomes Students work collaboratively, encouraging active involvement and participation and helping them to understand the subject more effectively. Building concept maps for any topic with a collaborative approach helps combine all students' knowledge, skills, and viewpoints into a complete and meaningful portrayal of the topic (Slieman and Camarata 2019). This approach will lead the students into critical thinking, analyzing information, and relating concepts.

Diverse Perspectives A significant characteristic of learning through collaboration is the opportunity for students to work with various learners from different backgrounds and with different perspectives (Slieman and Camarata 2019). Through teamwork, diverse experiences and views from other students are available, adding nuance to a topic. This diversity enriches the concept mapping process by introducing various modes of thought and approaches to problems and creatively and innovatively finding solutions.

Shared Knowledge and Resources A collaborative learning environment allows the sharing of knowledge, resources, and expertise between members. Students can draw on each other's strengths or forms of expertise to develop a higher-quality concept map (Slieman and Camarata 2019). Through shared ideas and collaboration, students have broader access to information through diversified perspectives, culminating in more holistic and detailed concept maps.

Collaboration promotes peer learning and support since students present complex concepts, clarify misconceptions, and offer support when needed. Working in groups further enhances friendship and closer associations among the students, providing them with a positive learning environment where they all value and support one another in their learning experiences.

Critical Thinking Development Collaborative learning environments are ideal for developing critical thinking skills such as problem-solving, analysis, and evaluation. Peer debate, discussion, and idea exchange lead students to critically appraise information and multiple viewpoints when making decisions (Slieman and Camarata 2019). Such critical thinking skills are indispensable for success in education and continued learning.

13.4.5 Interdisciplinary Collaboration and Effective Communication

Concept mapping helps cultivate essential skills, such as interdisciplinary collaboration and effective communication, in students through the collaborative development of concept maps.

The interdisciplinary nature of concept maps often involves combined knowledge from diverse disciplines or subject areas so that students can contribute to collaborative concept mapping using their expertise. Therefore, it is possible for students to understand how concepts created within different disciplines are interrelated and interact (Wang 2024). Additionally, this allows them to work on interdisciplinary issues that characterize future professional scenarios because collaboration across diverse fields with common interests is crucial.

Concept mapping is a collaborative effort that will be effective only if the members communicate well. To ensure that the concept map is meaningful and straightforward, students should present their views, provide feedback, and discuss their ideas with other group members (Wang 2024). In doing so, student members develop written and verbal communication skills, such as active listening, the ability to explain concepts, and the ability to share their opinions diplomatically. Proper, effective communication is vital for successful collaboration and is a skill one can take into the real world or apply in everyday life.

Conflicts or differences of opinion between the group members regarding the structure and content of the concept map may develop within the collaborative environment. Thus, students will have to apply effective strategies for conflict resolution—negotiation, compromise, and consensus building. Learning to navigate and resolve conflicts constructively enhances students' interpersonal skills and prepares them for effective teamwork on diverse teams.

Leadership and Followership Creating concept maps presents leadership opportunities. Individuals can demonstrate their skills in a leadership position or learn to be good followers while working in the group. A student can practice leadership by delegating some responsibilities, coordinating work performance, and motivating others on the team. Similarly, followership abilities can be enhanced by supporting group intentions, making proposals, and following the instructions given by the group leader (Wang 2024). Thus, both leadership and followership are effective team characteristics.

13.5 Summary and Conclusion

Concept mapping is an educational technique that is beneficial to health profession students since it provides a visual method that is structured for the organization and presentation of knowledge. This essay explains concept maps' essential elements in healthcare education: increasing ease in assessment and collaborative learning. Active learning, critical thinking, and long-term storage are encouraged when conceiving an arrangement of concepts in which learners may express their understanding of the relationships between various ideas and quickly identify gaps in knowledge. These maps are also effective in assessment and evaluation, as educators can effectively determine the level of students' understanding. The development of maps collaboratively also promotes teamwork, communication, and collaboration across disciplines. Thus, concept mapping improves learning and invigorates skills relevant to learners' healthcare practice.

References

Baliga SS, Walvekar PR, Mahantshetti GJ. Concept map as a teaching and learning tool for medical students. J Educ Health Promot. 2021;10:35.

Eachempati P, Ramnarayan K, Kiran Kumar KS, Mayya A. Concept maps for teaching, training, testing and thinking. MedEdPublish (2016). 2020;9:171.

Fonseca M, Marvão P, Oliveira B, Heleno B, Carreiro-Martins P, Neuparth N, Rendas A. The effectiveness of concept mapping as a tool for developing critical thinking in undergraduate medical education – a BEME systematic review: BEME Guide No. 81. Med Teach. 2023;46:1120–33.

Interaction Design Foundation. What are concept maps? — updated 2024. 2016. https://www.interaction-design.org/literature/topics/concept-maps#what_are_concept_maps?-0.

Joshi R, Hadley D, Nuthikattu S, Fok S, Goldbloom-Helzner L, Curtis M. Concept mapping as a metacognition tool in a problem-solving-based BME course during in-person and online instruction. Biomed Eng Educ. 2022;2:281–303.

Ligita T, Nurjannah I, Wicking K, Harvey N, Francis K. From textual to visual: the use of concept mapping as an analytical tool in a grounded theory study. Qual Res. 2020;22:126–42.

Mende S, Proske A, Narciss S. Individual preparation for collaborative learning: systematic review and synthesis. Educ Psychol. 2020;56:29–53.

Nicoara S-M, Szamoskozi S-E, Mitrea D-A, Leucuta D-C. Concept mapping, an effective tool for long-term memorization of anatomy-a quasi-experimental research carried out among 1st year general medicine students. Eur J Invest Health Psychol Edu. 2020;10:530–43.

Slieman TA, Camarata T. Case-based group learning using concept maps to achieve multiple educational objectives and behavioral outcomes. J Med Educ Curri Dev. 2019;6:2382120519872510.

Tarım SL, Boy Y, Şanlıtürk D. Effectiveness of the concept map in nursing education; developing a tool for student opinions. Hosp Pract Res. 2022;7:69–76.

Wang CC. Using design thinking for interdisciplinary curriculum design and teaching: a case study in higher education. Humanit Soc Sci Commun. 2024;11:179.

Coping with Stress in the Context of Education in the Health Professions

14

Khalid A. Bin Abdulrahman, Saleh Ahmed Alghamdi, and Eman Abdulkareem Abahussain

Learning Objectives

1. Identify the causes and manifestations of stress in health professions education, including academic, clinical, financial, and sociocultural factors.
2. Analyze the psychological, physical, and interpersonal effects of stress on students in health professions and recognize the characteristics of a stressed medical student.
3. Apply effective coping strategies, such as time management, self-care, mindfulness, and cognitive behavioral techniques, to mitigate stress and enhance well-being and academic performance.

14.1 Introduction

Stress is a normal physiological response to everyday obstacles and challenging circumstances; while it serves as an adaptive response, it may also become detrimental when it interferes with routine functioning. According to Vaishnavi (2023), stress triggers the body to release stress hormones such as cortisol and adrenaline, which prepare an individual for action both physically and biologically by increasing that individual's heart and

K. A. Bin Abdulrahman (✉)
Department of Medical Education, College of Medicine, Imam Mohammad Ibn Saud Islamic University (IMSIU), Riyadh, Saudi Arabia
e-mail: kab@imamu.edu.sa

S. A. Alghamdi · E. A. Abahussain
Department of Psychiatry, College of Medicine, Imam Mohammad Ibn Saud Islamic University (IMSIU), Riyadh, Saudi Arabia
e-mail: Saalghamedi@imamu.edu.sa; eabahussain@imamu.edu.sa

K. A. Bin Abdulrahman, H. Darami (eds.), *Essential Learning Skills for Health Professions Students*, https://doi.org/10.1007/978-981-96-5670-7_14

respiratory rates and fostering a state of attentiveness. Education in the health professions is challenging and entails a prolonged process. Students must complete many rigorous programs and courses that can equip them for subsequent employment in health professions. These programs entail both theoretical and clinical aspects, which, in combination with the process of learning and working in a competitive, complex, and demanding setting, can increase students' mental and physical stress, ultimately leading to a state of stress. This multilevel conception of stress in the context of education in the health professions requires an equally comprehensive approach to the task of managing such stress (Da Silva et al. 2021). Therefore, the health education system must play a pivotal role in the process of integrating stress management skills into professional education with the goals of supporting and enhancing the performance of health professionals.

14.2 Causes of Stress in the Context of Education in the Health Professions

14.2.1 High Expectations and Perfectionism

The field of healthcare both inspires individuals seeking to study medicine on the basis of its lofty standards and encouragement of a flawless approach and causes such individuals to experience stress. The eagerness of these individuals to reach or surpass such standards is often transformed to a self-driven demand to thrive in educational and clinical settings, which can result in apprehension about the possibility of failing to live up to the expected levels of proficiency. Perfectionism is a multifaceted personality characteristic that is associated with both beneficial and harmful subcategories. Henning and colleagues researched psychological adaptation among students from various health disciplines. These authors concluded that perfectionism and the impostor phenomenon (IP) were significant predictors of medical students' psychological discomfort (Henning et al. 1998).

Perfectionism encompasses a variety of characteristics, including a tendency to set excessively high objectives, engage in rigorous self-evaluations, establish unattainable standards for others, and harshly criticize those others. In light of these personality characteristics, success can become linked with feelings of anxiety and nervousness, and individuals can attribute their achievements to external factors such as luck. However, the temporary satisfaction resulting from these achievements fades as those individuals face the impending challenges, thereby perpetuating this cycle.

In fields that reward intellectual abilities, such as academia, imposter syndrome (according to which people believe they are undeserving of their successes despite objective evidence to the contrary) is common. IP has been reported to be prevalent at all hierarchical levels, ranging from novice students to seasoned surgeons, and exacerbate burnout among healthcare professionals, thus highlighting the importance of understanding this phenomenon.

Table 14.1 A summary of the causes of stress among health profession students and their key factors

Causes of stress	Key factors
High expectations and perfectionism	Pressure to meet high standards, perfectionism, and imposter syndrome
Clinical training	Long hours, high responsibility, exposure to suffering, and ethical dilemmas
Financial matters	High tuition costs, student debt, and financial strain
Personal life balance	Lack of time for personal life, social isolation, and health neglect
Transition to a professional role	Job uncertainties, professional demands, and imposter syndrome
Learning environment	Stressful teaching methods, inconsistent feedback, and lack of support
Sociocultural issues	Cultural, racial, and language barriers, along with parental expectations
Academic pressure	Intense curricula, high-stakes exams, and competitive programs

Individuals who are impacted by IP often develop distorted frames of reference for self-assessment, thus causing them to fail to recognize their successes internally, thereby impairing effective feedback processes.

However, the correlation between IP and perfectionism introduces another dimension to the processes of delivering or receiving criticism or feedback. Numerous studies have reported that IP and perfectionistic tendencies are noteworthy predictors of emotional turmoil among medical students and can cause individuals to be susceptible to various disorders, such as anxiety and depression. Table 14.1 provides a summary of the causes of stress among health profession students and their key factors.

14.2.2 Clinical Training

First, this context is characterized by a high level of responsibility. During clinical rotations, students are embedded in real-world healthcare settings and made accountable for patients, which can occasionally be challenging, particularly in severe or complex cases. Second, relevant problems in this context pertain to students' workload and hours. Students and trainees work the longest hours in this context, often including night and weekend shifts; this situation can lead to exhaustion and burnout. Third, the repetitive exposure of trainee doctors to human suffering, death, and ethical dilemmas leads to emotional stress.

14.2.3 Financial Matters

First, living expenses—including the need to establish a balance between the cost of living and books—exacerbate financial strain in this context. Second, financial strain is exacerbated by opportunity costs, as lengthy educational programs delay the point when students begin to earn professional salaries. Third, tuition and fees pertaining to education in the health professions are very high, resulting in considerable student debt. The cost burden associated with education in the health professions is increasing (Webster and North 2022). More students are taking out student loans as tuition continues to rise and wages continue to stagnate. The spiral resulting from this situation represents a source of acute concern for various institutions and occupations.

Furthermore, Webster and North (2022) examined the relationships between educational debt among health professional students and various personal, professional, and psychological factors by conducting a study of 5-year postgraduates. Table 14.1 reveals that educational debt is the most common influence on these personal factors. Factors that were cited by more than 50% of the respondents in that study are as follows (in descending order): savings, housing, leisure, discretionary spending, and family planning.

14.2.4 Personal Life Balance

First, time management is challenging because study and clinical hours leave students with little time for their personal lives, enjoyment, or relaxation. Second, study-intensive schedules can reduce students' social time with their family and friends, thus leading to social isolation. The third aspect is health neglect, since stressful schedules result in insufficient sleep, diet, and exercise.

14.2.5 Transition to a Professional Role

First, uncertainty pertaining to jobs, responsibilities, and job stability can be stressful. Second, many students experience imposter syndrome; namely, they feel that they are unprepared for professional jobs and call their own abilities into question, which can lead to self-doubt or worry. Third, professional demands from peers, mentors, and the healthcare system can be overwhelming.

14.2.6 Learning Environment

First, traditional teaching emphasizes memorization and rote learning, which can be stressful and alienating. Second, inconsistent or harsh comments and performance assessments from instructors affect students' self-esteem and motivation. Third, students may experience stress as a result of inadequate support systems, such as a lack of counselling or academic assistance.

14.2.7 Factors Pertaining to Sociocultural Issues

Cultural, racial, or gender issues as well as language barriers may increase the amount of stress that students from various backgrounds experience. Furthermore, cultural differences in parental expectations regarding academic success and job possibilities can easily lead to pressure.

14.2.8 Academic Pressure

With regard to intense curricula, programs for health professionals are renowned for their rigorous coursework, which requires students to absorb and retain vast amounts of information within a significantly short timeframe. Melaku et al. (2015) reported that academic-related stressors are the primary cause of stress among students, followed by teaching- and learning-related stressors. High-stakes exams, alongside ongoing evaluations such as midterms, finals, and board exams, consistently place pressure on students to excel. The competitiveness of such programs, which are often linked with limited job placements, can exacerbate the stress resulting from students' efforts to excel.

14.3 Characteristics of a Stressed Medical Student

14.3.1 Academic Struggles

Decreased academic performance can result in deteriorating grades, failed exams, or poor performance despite students' best efforts. The disproportionate pressure associated with medical education drives students toward social clashes that are characterized by decreased attention, low levels of mindfulness, reduced neutrality, increased chances of errors, and misbehavior, including negligence, thereby ultimately reducing their academic performance. Procrastination involves delaying assignments, studying, or the performance of one's clinical duties as a result of the feeling that one is overwhelmed.

14.3.2 Emotional Symptoms

Depression involves feelings of hopelessness, helplessness, and sadness as well as a loss of interest in activities that one has previously enjoyed. Mood swings refer to frequent changes in mood, ranging from anger to depression and frustration. Students may also experience anxiety and worry with regard to their performance in their studies, their future careers, or at the clinical level. Picton et al. (2022) posited that mental well-being deteriorates after learners are admitted to medical colleges. Mental health remains poor during the training process. Additionally, the environment that characterizes many medical schools involves pressure, particularly on the basis of a rigid and authoritative system that encourages competition among learners rather than cooperation (Gruyal et al. 2020). Such stress can persist throughout the internship period and individuals' postgraduate studies, ultimately impacting their careers as physicians.

14.3.3 Physical Symptoms

Students may experience sleep disturbances, such as poor sleep and frequently waking up, thereby generally affecting their rest. They may suffer from headaches and muscle tension, including neck pains, frequent headaches, and back pain resulting from physical and mental stress. Fatigue involves prolonged tiredness as a result of working long hours without adequate rest. Even after individuals receive sufficient sleep, they may continue to exhibit extreme tiredness. Medical students must understand the various dimensions of distress, such as total fatigue, that may be associated with their study schedules (Khosravi 2023). Students require an appropriate amount of sleep to address everyday activities and absorb information.

14.3.4 Interpersonal Relationships

Evidence of conflict with peers and supervisors can increase students' tension and conflict with their colleagues, instructors, and clinical supervisors. Decreased communication can cause them to lose interest in communicating freely and effectively with their fellows and mentors. Finally, in terms of strained family relations, students may be unable to maintain healthy relationships with their family members due to the time crunch and high levels of stress that they face.

14.3.5 Behavioral Changes

Isolation refers to a tendency to withdraw from social activities, family, and friends as a result of lack of time or emotional exhaustion. Students may also neglect personal care by exhibiting poor hygiene, failing to exercise, and developing unhealthy eating habits. They may engage in substance use, which involves the use of alcohol, caffeine, and drugs to cope with stress and anxiety. Melaku et al. (2015) reported that long-term stress negatively affects medical students' academic performance and is associated with substance use, depression, and suicide.

14.3.6 Cognitive Difficulties

Students can experience difficulty in making decisions; that is, as a result of excessive stress, they may not have the potential to make such decisions, or their decisions may be delayed. Inadequate problem-solving skills, which prevent students from thinking clearly and logically, can also cause issues with respect to students' academic and clinical performance. Students may also exhibit a loss of concentration, such that they are unable to focus in class, while studying, or while performing clinical work. Furthermore, they may experience memory problems forgetting important information, appointments, or clinical procedures. A small amount of stress can serve as a valuable catalyst for students, such as when anxiety regarding an upcoming exam inspires them to study. When such stress continues to accumulate, however, it might result in obstacles instead of benefits, thus increasing the difficulty of learning.

14.4 Strategies for Coping with Stress in the Context of Health Professions

14.4.1 Time Management

Time management techniques can help reduce stress among students. Yener et al. (2021) claimed that training programs pertaining to time management can reduce anxiety and enhance perceived control over time among students, thereby decreasing their stress. In particular, for nursing students, time management skills are beneficial because higher levels of time management are associated with lower levels of stress and improved academic performance. Several time management strategies can help reduce stress levels in the context of education in the health professions.

Tools such as lists, planners, and digital apps should be used to organize tasks. Individuals should prioritize tasks on the basis of their nature and focus on the most important tasks. Individuals can also set realistic goals by dividing large projects into small, manageable parts and then basing their goals on these smaller tasks, which can be completed on a daily or weekly basis. Students should schedule small breaks during their study sessions as well as larger breaks on a weekly basis to refresh themselves and prevent burnout. Overall, time management principles can effectively reduce stress in the lives of students and improve their well-being.

14.4.2 Mindfulness and Relaxation Techniques

Health professionals should practice mindfulness meditation to enhance their relaxation and enable them to focus and reduce stress. Online applications can help beginners in this regard. Engagement in progressive muscle relaxation exercises can help health professionals reduce physical tension and stress. Deep breathing exercises can also be used to manage acute stress and promote calmness during stressful situations.

14.4.3 Self-Care Practices

Individuals should exhibit a balanced diet by eating regular, balanced meals and remaining hydrated with the goal of supporting their physical and mental well-being. Health professionals should aim to attain adequate sleep, i.e., approximately 7 hours of sleep every night, to increase their cognitive function, improve their mood, and feel better during their daily lives. Individuals should engage in regular exercise by performing physical activities on a daily basis, including by walking, doing yoga, or visiting the gym. These activities can help reduce stress and improve individuals' overall health.

14.4.4 Social Support

Professionals should join or establish peer support groups to share their experiences, ask for advice, and provide mutual encouragement. In terms of connectedness, individuals must acquire the habit of contacting friends and family members frequently to receive emotional support from such individuals and to provide them with such support reciprocally.

14.4.5 Professional Support

In terms of counselling services, management should provide institutional mental health counselling services to enable students to cope with stress, anxiety, and mental illness. With regard to academic support, medical students should seek the help of academic advisors or tutors to improve their learning skills, enable them to handle the workload they face, and attain higher levels of academic performance. In terms of mental health, professionals should have mentors or individuals who can guide and help them search for answers to both academic and clinical problems. Wellness programs—i.e., well-being programs offered by the institution, such as workshops focusing on stress management and health promotion activities—are also essential in this context.

14.4.6 Cognitive Behavioral Strategies

With regard to positive self-talk, medical students should counteract negative thoughts by focusing on positive affirmations and more realistic views. In terms of goal setting, students should ensure that these goals are specific, measurable, attainable, relevant, and time-bound so that they can provide a satisfactory sense of accomplishment or direction in this regard. With respect to problem-solving skills, students should develop effective problem-solving skills to address academic and clinical issues systematically.

14.4.7 Balance and Boundaries

Work–life balance refers to efforts to establish a balance among academic responsibilities, personal interests, and leisure; such balance can help individuals minimize their levels of stress. To set boundaries, medical students should learn how to say no and divide their time appropriately while avoiding overcommitment. With regard to the topic of engagement in hobbies, medical students should not forget to indulge in pleasurable hobbies or leisure activities, such as reading, art, or sports, which could enable them to relax.

14.4.8 Healthy Coping Mechanisms

Journaling, i.e., keeping a journal, helps individuals reflect on the daily events of their lives, their feelings concerning those events, and the factors that cause stress. Such a journal represents a clearinghouse for thoughts and ideas, and stress can be alleviated when those thoughts and ideas are put into writing. Creative outlets—i.e., engaging in creative activities such as drawing, painting, or playing any instrument with the goals of venting one's emotions and unwinding—are necessary. Medical students who perform volunteer work can engage in volunteer activities or community services to obtain a novel perspective while simultaneously being able to give back and craft a sense of purpose.

14.4.9 Academic Strategies

Active learning includes strategies such as group studies, discussions, and teaching, and it can improve students' understanding and retentive power. Effective studying techniques among medical students can include spaced repetition, mnemonic devices, and information summaries to increase the efficiency of learning. In terms of resources, medical students should use academic resources that are made available to them, such as online courses, textbooks, and practice exams, to supplement their learning. Table 14.2 summarizes the strategies for coping with stress in health professions.

In summary, stress in the context of education in the health professions is the result of academic, clinical, economic, personal, professional, environmental, and social factors. Addressing these causal variables requires a strategy that encompasses academic assistance, mental health services, financial support, and the enhancement of both work–life balance and resilience. Understanding and alleviating these pressures can empower educational institutions to help learners manage and achieve success during their training and

Table 14.2 A summary of the strategies used for coping with stress in health professions

Strategies	Key approaches
Time management	Use tools like planners, prioritize tasks, and schedule breaks
Mindfulness and relaxation techniques	Practice mindfulness meditation, deep breathing, and relaxation exercises
Self-care practices	Maintain a balanced diet, engage in regular exercise, and ensure adequate sleep
Social support	Join peer support groups and maintain strong connections with family and friends
Professional support	Seek counseling, academic advisors, and participate in wellness programs
Cognitive behavioral strategies	Use positive self-talk, set realistic goals, and enhance problem-solving skills
Balance and boundaries	Establish work–life balance, set boundaries, and engage in hobbies
Healthy coping mechanisms	Practice journaling, engage in creative activities, and participate in volunteer work
Academic strategies	Adopt active learning techniques and utilize academic resources

their subsequent professional lives. Recognizing the characteristics of a stressed medical student is crucial with respect to efforts to provide such students with prompt support and interventions. Establishing comprehensive support systems and facilitating the emergence of a healthy equilibrium among the academic, clinical, and personal aspects that are typically associated with professional education, such as medicine, could significantly alleviate stress and enhance the well-being and performance exhibited by medical students. The task of managing stress in the context of education in the health professions encompasses various strategies that integrate effective time management with self-care, mindfulness, social support, consulting, cognitive behavioral techniques, balance, and healthy coping mechanisms. In this manner, a student can deal effectively with stress, exhibit improved well-being, and become successful at both the academic and professional levels.

References

Da Silva ATC, De Souza Lopes C, Susser E, Coutinho LMS, Germani ACCG, Menezes PR. Burnout among primary health care workers in Brazil: results of a multilevel analysis. Int Arch Occup Environ Health. 2021;94:1863–75.

Gruyal HAA, Madiam PEI, Gregorio MAO, Magsombol MEH, Guanzon AAO, Magtibay MTLH. Association of extracurricular activities on academic stress of medical students: a cross-sectional study. Int J Stud Educ Sci (IJSES). 2020;1:92–111.

Henning K, Ey S, Shaw D. Perfectionism, the impostor phenomenon and psychological adjustment in medical, dental, nursing and pharmacy students. Med Educ. 1998;32:456–64.

Khosravi M. Factors affecting medical students' academic burnout: a moderation analysis. Ital J Med. 2023;17:1659.

Melaku L, Mossie A, Negash A. Stress among medical students and its association with substance use and academic performance. J Biomed Educ. 2015;2015:1–9.
Picton A, Greenfield S, Parry J. Why do students struggle in their first year of medical school? A qualitative study of student voices. BMC Med Educ. 2022;22:100.
Vaishnavi H. The secrets to live a stress-free life: an ultimate roadmap to eliminate stress and heal your mind. Chhattisgarh: Shashwat Publication; 2023.
Webster P, North SE. Health professions educational debt: personal, professional, and psychological impacts 5 years post-graduation. Front Med. 2022;9:746463.
Yener S, Arslan A, Kilinç S. The moderating roles of technological self-efficacy and time management in the technostress and employee performance relationship through burnout. Inf Technol People. 2021;34(7):1890–919.

Further Reading

Bynum WE, Artino AR, Uijtdehaage S, Webb AMB, Varpio L. Sentinel emotional events: the nature, triggers, and effects of shame experiences in medical residents. Acad Med. 2019;94:85–93.
Clance PR, Dingman D, Reviere SL, Stober DR. Impostor phenomenon in an interpersonal/social context. Women Ther. 1995;16:79–96.
Everyday Health. Health impacts: exercise and stress relief. 2024. Available from https://www.everydayhealth.com/exercise-photos/exercises-that-relieve-stress.aspx.
Franchi T, Russell-Sewell N. Medical students and the impostor phenomenon: a coexistence precipitated and perpetuated by the educational environment? Med Sci Educ. 2022;33:27–38.
Hewitt PL, Flett GL. Perfectionism in the self and social contexts: conceptualization, assessment, and association with psychopathology. J Pers Soc Psychol. 1991;60:456–70.
Hutchins HM. Outing the imposter: a study exploring imposter phenomenon among higher education faculty. New Horiz Adult Educ Hum Resour Dev. 2015;27:3–12.
Moridi G, Khaledi S, Valiee S. Clinical training stress-inducing factors from the students' viewpoint: A questionnaire-based study. Nurse Educ Pract. 2014;14:160–3.
Rohrmann S, Bechtoldt MN, Leonhardt M. Validation of the impostor phenomenon among managers. Front Psychol. 2016;7:821.
Thomas M, Bigatti S. Perfectionism, impostor phenomenon, and mental health in medicine: a literature review. Int J Med Educ. 2020;11:201–13.
Yu JH, Chae SJ, Chang KH. The relationship among self-efficacy, perfectionism and academic burnout in medical school students. Korean J Med Educ. 2016;28:49–55.

15 Students' Perspectives on the Pros and Cons of Current Instructional and Learning Methods

Amro Khalid Bin Abdulrahman and Hamad Saleh Alturki

Learning Objectives

1. *Analyse the pros and cons of instructional methods.*
   - Evaluate the advantages and limitations of various instructional methods such as problem-based learning (PBL), active learning, and the integration of basic and clinical phases, focusing on their impact on student learning outcomes and professional development.
2. *Understand the role of holistic learning environments.*
   - Explore the significance of student-teacher relationships, extracurricular activities, and community engagement in fostering a supportive, engaging, and effective educational atmosphere for medical and health students.
3. *Identify strategies to address psychological and academic challenges.*
   - Recognise the factors contributing to psychological pressures, burnout, and stress in medical education and propose strategies, such as mindfulness techniques, mentorship programs, and balanced assessment tools, to enhance student well-being and academic performance.

The original version of the chapter has been revised. A correction to this chapter can be found at https://doi.org/10.1007/978-981-96-5670-7_16

A. K. Bin Abdulrahman (✉)
Senior Registrar and Preventive Medicine Specialist, Alumni of the College of Medicine, Imam Mohammad Ibn Saud Islamic University (IMSIU), Department of Preventive Medicine, Second Cluster, Ministry of Health, Riyadh, Saudi Arabia
e-mail: draka.1416@gmail.com

H. S. Alturki
Alumni of College of Medicine, Imam Mohammad Ibn Saud Islamic University (IMSIU), Healthcare Leadership Academy at the Saudi Commission for Health Specialties, Riyadh, Saudi Arabia
e-mail: alturki.hamad1@gmail.com

K. A. Bin Abdulrahman, H. Darami (eds.), *Essential Learning Skills for Health Professions Students*, https://doi.org/10.1007/978-981-96-5670-7_15

15.1 Introduction

The current educational industry is characterised by its dynamism, which exposes students to a diverse array of instructional and learning techniques. The wide range of instructional methods is rooted in the need for educators to optimise the offerings provided to students. In addition, the consistently evolving learning environment dictates that no single instructional method is suitable for all students and all learning conditions. Therefore, students' perspectives on a variety of instructional and learning methods have proven valuable, as the students are the main beneficiaries of these techniques. Positive improvements in performance are observed when an instructional or learning method is suitable for the students' needs. This observation is also true for instructional methods that might lead to unfavourable outcomes in different areas of learning. To better understand the advantages and disadvantages associated with various techniques, students' perspectives and inputs are necessary, given the critical role they play in improving the techniques. Additionally, students have a chance to propose potential modifications that could achieve greater outcomes from different learning methods. Various instructional and learning methodologies have been implemented in medical and health institutions to facilitate the acquisition and dissemination of knowledge. The perspectives of students on modern learning techniques, such as the relationship between the student and the teacher, the integration of the basic medical phase with the clinical phase, and the use of problem-based learning, are the focus of this chapter. The findings may prove essential in identifying the advantages and disadvantages of different instructional methods and in determining how to address those disadvantages to better suit the needs of medical and health college students.

15.1.1 Problem-Based Learning (PBL)

In modern medical and health college settings, PBL is one of the most prevalent techniques. The foundations of PBL are distinct from those of traditional teaching methods, which entail the complete control of the learning process by the teacher (Ali et al. 2024). Instead, PBL recognises students as the focal point of their educational experience. In other words, PBL encourages students to drive the learning process through the exploration of real-world medical problems. The method enables learners to establish personal objectives, identify needs, and conduct independent research. Additionally, this method facilitates collaboration between learners to resolve various kinds of problems (Páez et al. 2024). In the context of PBL, learners are not merely passive participants in the learning process; rather, they actively utilise lifelong attributes, such as critical thinking, research, discussion, communication, collaboration, and problem-solving, which are essential for the professional development of future medical professionals (Alexander et al. 2024).

Various advantages are associated with PBL from the students' perspective. PBL enables students to develop a deeper understanding of the subject matter. As previously mentioned, PBL enables students to construct real-world scenarios that correspond to the theoretical concepts they have acquired in class (Chang 2023). Additionally, students can develop critical thinking skills and innovative solutions to a variety of challenges using PBL. On a personal note, I vividly recall the discussions from the PBL sessions. My colleagues and I were actively immersed in these interactions, which improved our understanding and retention of information. I consider the experience of identifying gaps in the case and investigating various solutions to address these gaps to be valuable components of my professional growth as a health practitioner.

Currently, it is imperative for health practitioners to develop effective communication skills in clinical settings, and PBL can significantly improve these skills (Leszczyński et al. 2018). Some students will concentrate predominantly on the academic and knowledge aspects, without giving much attention to essential skills that will improve their communication within clinical settings, which plays a major role in improving patient outcomes (Sany et al. 2020). Consequently, collaborative discussions and communication in PBL are vital for achieving success as healthcare professionals. This development is facilitated by a variety of perspectives, such as interpersonal and cross-cultural communication. This type of communication is important because healthcare is currently characterised by cultural diversity, which may impede the comprehension of professionals with limited communication skills (Kerimbayev et al. 2023). Overall, PBL is an essential instrument for cultivating lifelong learning abilities. PBL has demonstrated an ability to promote self-directed learning, making it a critical instrument for the development of skills that enable learners to remain informed about the ever-changing medical field.

Although PBL has the benefits described above, there are also numerous disadvantages from the viewpoint of the students that need to be addressed. Initially, the exclusive implementation of PBL can be time-consuming. For example, implementing PBL involves independent learning or case studies that require students to delve more thoroughly into unfamiliar subjects. Compared with teacher-led instruction, independent learning may require more time to complete. Another disadvantage of PBL is that facilitators may find it difficult to grasp the expectations placed on them (Leszczyński et al. 2018). Faculty development and training in facilitation are essential for the successful implementation of PBL. However, some institutions do not regard facilitation as an essential part of PBL, even though students are susceptible to confusion in their attempts to identify and complete specific objectives in the absence of facilitation (Alexander et al. 2024). Even when facilitation is provided, both underfacilitation, which could result in confusion, and overfacilitation, which could transform the PBL session into a lecture, are possible. Another drawback of PBL is the greater workload that students are required to take on since this method is centred on them. Therefore, the approach requires that students be adequately equipped to engage in and make significant contributions during PBL sessions. Additionally, some institutions allocate minimal weight to PBL grades, which may lead to students neglecting these activities in favour of assignments or exams of higher weight. Thus, it is advisable to give PBL assignments more weight or making them a requirement for passing the course. This approach would motivate students to prepare thoroughly and push themselves beyond their comfort zones, whether in discussions or learning with diverse groups.

Table 15.1 Pros and cons of problem-based learning (PBL) from students' perspective

Pros	Cons
Student-centred learning approach	Time-consuming process
Encourages critical thinking and problem-solving	Requires experienced facilitators
Develops lifelong skills, such as collaboration and communication	High workload for students
Facilitates application of theoretical concepts to real-world scenarios	Potential for uneven participation among students
Promotes self-directed learning	Challenges in assessment and evaluation

In other words, PBL has potential value as an essential learning method in the field of modern healthcare. However, it is necessary to analyse several of the shortcomings of its implementation. The advantages and disadvantages of PBL are summarised in Table 15.1.

15.1.2 Integration of Basic Medical Phases and the Clinical Phase

Modern educational approaches necessitate early introduction to the clinical stages of learning. In the early years of medical and health institutions, a substantial amount of attention was directed towards enabling students to grasp the scientific foundations of diverse concepts (Al-Zahrani 2024). Clinical practice was eventually introduced to students at the later phases of their education. The traditional pedagogical methods proved insufficient, failing to facilitate the application of knowledge acquired in the classroom to real-world clinical environments. Furthermore, the students required extended transitional periods to align with the constantly changing conditions in clinical environments. Consequently, integration of the foundational and clinical phases has been established to facilitate a more pertinent connection between academic instruction and practical applications (Kerimbayev et al. 2023). When early clinical experiences are meticulously organised, closely monitored, and customised to align with different learning phases, these students are likely to navigate different areas of medical and health education with improved efficacy.

From the perspective of the student, integrating the basic medical and clinical stages offers both significant benefits and drawbacks. This method offers the benefit of early immersion in the clinical environment (Al-Zahrani 2024). The integration of basic and clinical phases facilitates students' capacity to effectively and swiftly translate the theories acquired in the classroom into practical applications in clinical settings. This approach enables students to gain insight into their strengths and weaknesses across different learning domains. When performed with care, this method has the potential to guide students in improving their strengths while concurrently addressing specific weaknesses (Kerimbayev et al. 2023). The second benefit associated with this method is the facilitation of learning continuity. The integration facilitates fluid progression across different phases of learning,

Table 15.2 Pros and cons of integration between the basic medical and clinical phases from students' perspective

Pros	Cons
Early exposure to clinical environments	Complex curriculum design and implementation
Facilitates seamless learning continuity	Resource-intensive process
Increases student motivation and engagement	Logistical challenges in execution
Enhances application of theoretical knowledge to practice	Requires continuous supervision and monitoring

cultivating a more integrated educational experience for the students. Moreover, students in health and medical fields often find greater engagement through practical and experiential learning opportunities. Initial engagement with practical or clinical skills inspires students to deepen their understanding and fully grasp the relationships between foundational knowledge and clinical application. Furthermore, the incorporation of practical applications prompts students to engage in simulations of real-world scenarios, thus improving educational methodologies through application, discussion, and various interactive approaches.

Despite these described benefits, integration may also present a range of disadvantages. Primarily, there may be complexities linked to integration in some situations. Some students may encounter difficulties with the learning curve, which requires the application of theoretical knowledge within clinical environments (Atashinsadaf et al. 2024). To mitigate the stress and complexity associated with this integration, it is imperative to thoroughly evaluate logistics and faculty workloads to facilitate seamless integration. Furthermore, initial clinical experiences should be thoroughly structured, closely monitored, and customised to align with the learner's learning stage. Another drawback linked to this approach is the requirement for substantial resources for its successful implementation. Successful integration of the learning phases necessitates the provision of resources, particularly facilitators with requirements for quantity and calibre. Furthermore, institutions may require additional resources to facilitate access to clinical settings (Chang et al. 2023). If not managed effectively, the integration process may consume additional resources, thereby depriving other essential departments within the institutions.

Table 15.2 summarises the pros and cons of integration between the basic medical phase and clinical phase.

15.1.3 Educational Environment that Stimulates Active Learning

The methodologies cultivated within the educational environment can significantly influence the extent of knowledge and skills that students acquire. Active learning is a method that has been promoted in various medical and health education settings

(Rozhenkova et al. 2023). Active learning encompasses techniques that guide students in actively participating in their educational journeys. Some of the techniques utilised in active learning are retrieval-based strategies, interleaving, and spacing. Research has demonstrated that students who pursue undergraduate degrees in STEM fields are at a disadvantage if they are predominantly exposed to lecture formats. Compared with their peers, students exhibit a fivefold greater likelihood of failing their exams in courses that integrate active learning techniques (Bose et al. 2024). Active learning cultivates an environment that is both secure and stimulating, fostering the growth and development of students. Through active engagement with their peers and instructors, students frequently find themselves inspired by the depth of discussions. The combination of various cognitive approaches and analytical frameworks facilitates a rich learning environment, allowing each student to benefit from the insights of their peers. This interaction fosters retention and deep understanding, encouraging students to engage in further learning activities in both the short and long term.

However, active learning has several disadvantages that medical institutions and their stakeholders need to consider. A notable challenge associated with this approach is assessment and evaluation (Rozhenkova et al. 2023). Given the focus on distinctive techniques tailored to each learner, evaluating students fairly can present significant challenges. I believe it would be best to incorporate some elements and techniques of active learning into the overall learning method rather than utilising active learning as the sole learning method. This incorporation can be achieved by instilling the ability to think scientifically and formulate effective academic discussions that meet assessment requirements in students. Knowledge and skills are improved and nourished over time, and understanding the methods and core principles of learning will enable students to excel and discover new, innovative ways to suit their individual needs and learning objectives. Active learning presents certain challenges in classroom management as well, as it necessitates the vigilant oversight of each learner's engagement. Medical students may also find active learning to be time-consuming, and the substantial workload may not align closely with the rigorous demands of the content-rich curriculums of health specialties. Table 15.3 summarises the pros and cons of active learning from healthcare students' perspective.

Table 15.3 Pros and cons of active learning from healthcare students' perspective

Pros	Cons
Encourages engagement and participation	Challenges in assessment and evaluation
Develops higher-order thinking skills	Classroom management can be complex
Improves retention and understanding of material	Time-consuming for both students and instructors
Promotes inclusivity and collaborative learning	Increased workload for students
Provides a safe and stimulating learning environment	Difficult to align with content-heavy curriculum

15.1.4 Relationship Between the Student and the Teacher

The relationship between students and teachers has been a significant factor in improving academic performance in various methods. To cultivate a robust educational atmosphere, some institutions prioritise positive and encouraging relationships between teachers and students (Bose et al. 2024). Students tend to achieve greater success and increased satisfaction when they are surrounded by teachers with whom they can interact openly. Success may be contingent upon multiple factors. Primarily, the majority of student learning activities continue to be dependent on the acquisition of knowledge from teachers (Shrivastava and Shrivastava 2021). Consequently, when students experience a sense of ease in engaging with faculty, they are more inclined to seek clarification or ask questions that are crucial to their academic growth. Furthermore, the development of positive rapport between instructors and students can contribute to the improvement of instructional and learning methods. Consider, for example, the PBL method, which necessitates that teachers support the learning experience. In the absence of a positive relationship, a teacher may find it difficult to guide students in recognising their strengths and weaknesses or establishing specific goals (Abuhassna et al. 2024).

Student-teacher relationships that are constructive promote growth for both the faculty and the students. For example, teachers can offer a safe environment while motivating students to venture beyond their comfort zones, acquire new skills, and establish a mentoring network. Students are more likely to seek out and receive assistance, guidance, and mentorship from their teachers when they have a positive connection with them (Jebreen et al. 2024). For a student, this relationship facilitates opportunities for engagement, which is essential to the educational experience.

However, the effect of the teacher-student relationship on power dynamics is one of the known drawbacks. In most situations, the relationship between teachers and specific students might vary from one teacher to another or from one student to another. Consequently, these relationships are likely to spark bias, favouritism, or dishonesty in addressing different student needs (Darmawansah et al. 2023). Furthermore, the dynamics of these relationships may foster a sense of reliance; students may become overly dependent on the relationships they cultivate with their teachers, leading to an excessive reliance on the perspectives provided by those educators. An excessive reliance on the guidance of educators may also inhibit students' capacity to cultivate their independent learning skills.

Graph 1 illustrates the necessary balance that needs to be established between the students and the teachers.

15.1.5 Extracurricular Activities and Community Engagement

For medical and health students, the traditional emphasis on clinical rotations and extensive classroom instruction is rapidly shifting. Currently, institutions are placing greater

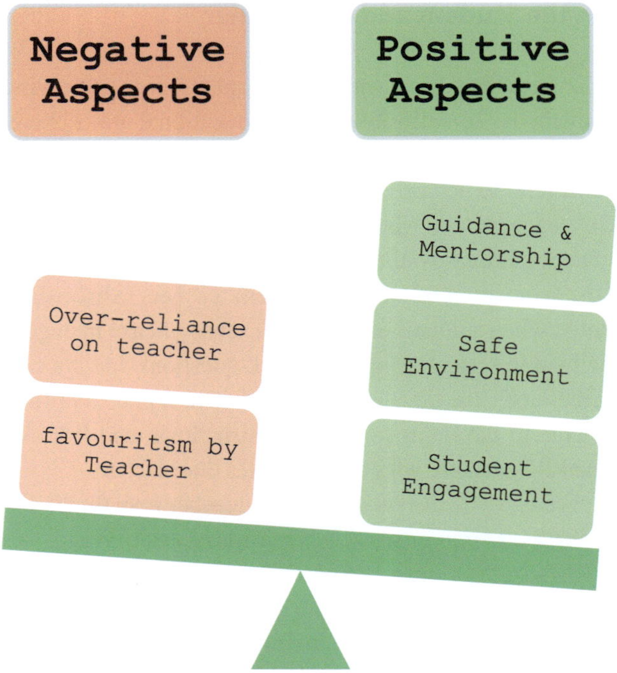

Graph 1

emphasis on extracurricular activities (ECAs) and community engagement initiatives (Leszczyński et al. 2018). Independent of their academic performance in the classroom, students' physical and cognitive health are improved through their involvement in ECAs and community engagement. The majority of colleges have created distinctive ECA and community engagement programs according to the requirements of their students. Health promotion events serve as community engagement initiatives through which students can interact with their local communities (Abuhassna et al. 2024). These events may encompass health conferences, seminars, or health education campaigns focused on disease prevention, nutrition, and physical exercise. Institutions may organise peer and near-peer tutoring and mentorship programs, enabling students to seek support and strengthen their foundations in areas such as leadership. Additional activities could involve engagement in physical activities, participation in research initiatives, volunteering at hospitals or clinics, and collaboration with professional organisations.

The suitability of ECAs and community engagement in students' education has been reviewed from different perspectives. According to Darmawansah et al. (Darmawansah et al. 2023), students benefit from participating in ECAs since they can utilise these opportunities to progress in other aspects of their education. For example, participating in sports and other physical activities helps students' psychological well-being, which is crucial for reducing stress and anxiety throughout the learning journey. Additionally, learners can broaden their knowledge by interacting with professionals from various sectors and fields. Third, volunteering in clinics or community awareness campaigns is a crucial activity for students because these programs introduce students to some of the real-life scenarios they could encounter as healthcare professionals (Rozhenkova et al. 2023). Nevertheless, it is imperative that institutions establish an appropriate balance between academic work and ECAs and community engagement programs. Excessive emphasis on programs or activities may result in certain learners neglecting their academic responsibilities. Furthermore, ECAs do not consistently benefit learners, as some activities may lack contributions to students' academic development. These issues may be resolved by designating specific times and weights for extracurricular activities within each course and by creating an ECA program that promotes student participation during the summer. During this time, students are usually more at ease and receptive to new challenges and educational opportunities. These kinds of activities can help students develop several areas of their personalities, increase their self-esteem and satisfaction, and assist them in earlier identification of their professional pathways.

Table 15.4 summarises the pros and cons of ECAs and community engagement.

15.1.6 Learning in the Simulation Centre Using Standardised Patients

The establishment of simulation centres that utilise standardised patients (SPs) is transforming healthcare education in numerous ways. Simulators are designed to present learners with a variety of case scenarios while minimising risk (Tefera et al. 2024). Simulation activities are typically performed in environments that replicate healthcare settings, enabling learners to engage in experiences reflective of their future professional roles. SPs are trained professionals capable of simulating patients exhibiting particular behaviours, emotions, and medical conditions. With the use of SPs and simulators, students can be exposed to a variety of situations in which they can connect to real-life scenarios (Rozhenkova et al. 2023). The learning process requires the SPs to adhere to predetermined scripts to guarantee an unbiased assessment of each student's performance. In certain situations, SPs may engage in simulation programs and respond to various enquiries posed by students during the learning process.

Simulators and SPs enable students to develop various competencies, including decision-making, communication, and clinical skills, in controlled and safe environments

Table 15.4 Pros and cons of extracurricular activities and community engagement from healthcare students' perspective

Pros	Cons
Promotes holistic development and personal growth	May impact academic performance if not balanced
Provides real-life exposure to healthcare scenarios	Unequal benefits depending on activity structure
Enhances leadership and mentorship skills	Can increase stress and pressure on students
Expands knowledge through diverse experiences	May conflict with other academic commitments
Improves physical and mental well-being	Potential financial costs for participation

Table 15.5 Pros and cons of learning in the simulation centre and using standardised patients from healthcare students' perspective

Pros	Cons
Provides a safe and controlled learning environment	High costs for maintenance and operation
Offers realistic clinical scenarios	Scenarios may feel artificial compared to real-world complexity
Enhances skill development in communication, decision-making, and clinical tasks	Limited exposure to the unpredictability of real clinical settings
Facilitates interactive and hands-on learning	Requires instructor expertise and resources
Allows objective evaluation and feedback	Overreliance on simulations may hinder empathy and adaptability with real patients

prior to interacting with actual patients (Boon 2024). This method diminishes student anxiety and increases confidence. Simulators and SPs can effectively improve competencies in communication, physical examination skills, and differential diagnoses, which are essential for learner development (Abuhassna et al. 2024). However, the maintenance of simulators and SPs can be costly for many institutions to sustain over time. Furthermore, owing to the artificial nature of these scenarios, students may not encounter the complexity and unpredictability inherent in actual clinical settings. Another drawback is that students may become overly dependent on simulations, which might hinder their communication skills and empathy towards real patients. Therefore, this method of instruction could gradually expose younger students to real-world situations that they might encounter in their future work.

Table 15.5 summarises the pros and cons of learning in the simulation centre and using SPs.

15.1.7 Assessment Tools

Numerous colleges and educational institutions in healthcare are shifting from traditional multiple-choice questions (MCQs) to more integrated assessment models. MCQs are frequently regarded as the standardised method for evaluating broad knowledge; however, they may not accurately represent clinical reasoning and decision-making skills in clinical environments (Tefera et al. 2024). Consequently, alternative assessment techniques are needed to offer a comprehensive perspective on students' performance that aligns more effectively with the current dynamic health sector (Boon 2024). One technique is the objective structured clinical examination (OSCE), which is used to evaluate clinical activities, including communication, history taking, and physical examination. Emerging techniques for assessing medical students include portfolio assessments, e-portfolios, and 360-degree evaluations. Each of these techniques can be applied on the basis of their suitability for the defined scenarios.

The incorporation of different assessment techniques has both positive and negative effects from the students' perspective. On the positive end, the different techniques exhibit a level of dynamism comparable to that of the clinical setting (Boon 2024). These assessments also address emerging clinical issues rather than relying on static conventional methods. Furthermore, the emphasis on evaluating skills, attitudes, and professional behaviours, rather than knowledge alone, has directed efforts towards the development of well-rounded professionals. Other techniques enhance clinical reasoning in learners by assessing their ability to apply the knowledge acquired in class to clinical settings. Additionally, the new techniques facilitate lifelong learning by utilising tools that emphasise self-reflection and portfolio assessments, enabling learners to achieve independence and self-reliance in acquiring and sharing knowledge (Kilipiris et al. 2024). On the other hand, developing and validating new assessment techniques is often time-consuming and requires significant resources. However, the utilisation of various resources in the development and implementation of techniques does not ensure their consistency and reliability. Moreover, educators require training for the successful implementation of these techniques. Nevertheless, employing multiple assessment tools is essential to ensure that students possess the necessary competencies to succeed as healthcare professionals.

Given that the primary objective of medical colleges is to produce safe doctors, some students argue that the implementation of a pass/fail assessment system, as opposed to relying solely on academic grades, could be beneficial in the evaluation of core competencies and critical learning outcomes. This approach may diminish the focus on attaining higher GPAs, which frequently cultivates excessive competitiveness. This competitiveness may hinder the learning experience by promoting individual achievement over peer support and potentially inducing excessive anxiety. In conclusion, any medical institution should strive to provide comprehensive assessment criteria that guarantee that students are attaining the desired competences and developing into safe health practitioners in a secure learning environment.

Table 15.6 summarises the pros and cons of the new student assessment tools and current examination status.

Table 15.6 Pros and cons of new student assessment tools and current examination status from healthcare students' perspective

Pros	Cons
Offers dynamic and realistic assessment methods	Development and implementation are time-consuming and resource-intensive
Provides holistic evaluation, including skills and attitudes	Consistency and reliability of tools may vary
Enhances clinical reasoning and problem-solving skills	Requires significant educator training
Reduces competitiveness, fostering a collaborative environment	Balancing knowledge-based and practical assessments can be challenging
Encourages lifelong learning through reflective tools like portfolios	May not fully align with traditional grading systems

15.1.8 Participation in Research and Scientific Publishing

Research and publishing serve as fundamental components of knowledge sharing in medical and health education. Facilitating student-led research studies improves knowledge across multiple learning domains (Boon 2024). In modern medical and health education, research and publishing can be facilitated through workshops focused on scientific writing, mentorship programs, and fellowships and grants. Participation in research and publication offers numerous benefits. For example, critical thinking can be improved through research or publication; specifically, learners can implement strategies to challenge assumptions, analyse data, become acquainted with scientific methodologies, and derive evidence-based findings from the results (Kilipiris et al. 2024). Additionally, developing research proposals can improve a student's communication ability. These proposals facilitate student engagement and collaboration with diverse stakeholders in research, including fellow researchers and Institutional Review Board committees. Students gain vital communication skills from these exchanges, such as how to effectively present their research. Students also acquire experience in grant applications and the management of research projects. Research and publication activities can improve students' comprehension of healthcare, increase their problem-solving skills, and allow them to recognise gaps in the literature while proposing innovative solutions to the scientific healthcare community.

However, students' perspectives indicate that there are some difficulties that need to be considered when incorporating research and publication techniques into education. First, the methods necessitate substantial faculty involvement; educational institutions should allocate additional resources to mentorship programs to guide students in effective research and publication strategies (Boon 2024). Research and publishing require significant resources and increased investment in operations such as data collection. Furthermore, scheduling medical and health programs can complicate the balance between these efforts and standard academic activities. Additionally, access to research and publishing programs is not uniformly available to all students. Consequently, programs may perpetuate bias if they are not designed equitably for all learners. The incorporation of research projects into the curriculum is one potential solution to these challenges. This method would motivate students to engage in research that aligns with their interests and to seek advice from faculty members or experts. A paper by Abdulrahman (2022) summarises the lessons learned from student research and presents strategies for addressing challenges in various aspects of health research.

Table 15.7 summarises the pros and cons of participation in research and scientific publishing.

Table 15.7 Pros and cons of participation in research projects and scientific publishing from healthcare students' perspective

Pros	Cons
Enhances critical thinking and analytical skills	Requires extensive faculty integration and mentorship
Improves writing and communication abilities	Resource-intensive process
Develops advanced understanding of healthcare topics	Balancing academic and research activities can be challenging
Provides opportunities for professional and career development	Access to research opportunities may not be equitable
Encourages collaboration and problem-solving	Potential bias if programs are not inclusive

15.1.9 Psychological Pressure and Educational Burnout

Students in health and medical institutions are developing in distinctive settings that may expose them to a variety of psychological pressures and educational burnout. The psychological pressures may be partially attributed to the high demand for success, emotional stress from clinical settings, and the intense educational requirements associated with continuous exams and assessments (Medeiros et al. 2024). In contrast, educational fatigue may result from emotional exhaustion, depersonalisation, and a diminished sense of accomplishment among students. Failures among students may result from any of the aforementioned psychological pressures and exhaustion factors. Fortunately, stakeholders in medical and health education institutions can adopt a variety of coping strategies to alleviate these effects (Wankhar et al. 2024). The initial approach should involve the establishment of support systems. To manage fatigue and stress, students in active environments require stable support systems, such as mental health services and peer and near-peer support groups. Second, providing students with exposure to a variety of essential skills is crucial; communication and time management skills can assist students in handling specific pressure-related difficulties (Xiao et al. 2024). Gradually, educational institutions may integrate mindfulness and relaxation strategies into their curricula. The techniques mentioned above are essential for assisting students in recognising their limitations and concentrating on a variety of factors that extend beyond academic success. It is imperative to offer mentorship from senior students and access to official mental health counsellors and provide workshops or seminars on the prevention of burnout, anxiety, and depression. These resources have the potential to substantially reduce stress, regardless of whether they are implemented through formal or informal programs. For example, students can learn that stress is a common occurrence and can be effectively managed. Students should also be instructed to report any instances in which burnout symptoms or social, mental, or physical issues have a significant impact on their lives. Students are also encouraged to seek the assistance of their mentors when they are feeling overworked.

Table 15.8 Pros and cons of psychological pressures and educational burnout from healthcare students' perspective

Pros	Cons
Encourages the development of coping skills	High academic demands can lead to stress and anxiety
Promotes the use of mindfulness and relaxation techniques	Emotional stress from clinical environments impacts performance
Builds resilience and adaptability	Reduced sense of accomplishment due to burnout
Supports the creation of mentorship and support systems	Peer pressure and unhealthy academic comparisons
Encourages a holistic view of health, including mental and emotional well-being	Grading systems can exacerbate stress and competitiveness

Students should embrace a comprehensive perspective on health, which includes physical, mental, social, and spiritual well-being. These interrelated elements help create a stable, well-rounded personality, which is essential for professional success. Furthermore, students should be encouraged to refrain from drawing comparisons with their classmates, acknowledging that each student has their own unique style and pace. As previously stated, the grading system can have a detrimental effect on some students, while others perceive grades as a substantial affirmation of their academic accomplishments and self-assurance. A pass/fail system could alleviate some of the anxiety associated with the competitive nature of applying to speciality programs that require high GPAs and exam scores while also fostering a safer environment for effective learning.

Table 15.8 summarises the pros and cons of psychological pressure and educational burnout.

15.2 Summary

This chapter explores students' perspectives on instructional methods in medical and health education, highlighting the importance of diverse approaches to meet evolving student needs. Key methods include problem-based learning, integration of medical and clinical phases, and active learning. Factors influencing student experiences include student-teacher relationships, extracurricular activities, assessment tools, and research participation. Balancing traditional and innovative methods is crucial for a supportive, adaptive educational environment. The insights aim to guide stakeholders in refining instructional strategies to improve outcomes and address diverse student needs.

References

Abdulrahman AKB. Student as a researcher: a perspective of a Saudi medical student. Int J Med Res Health Sci. 2022;11:1–8.

Abuhassna H, Adnan MABM, Awae F. Exploring the synergy between instructional design models and learning theories: a systematic literature review. Contemp Educ Technol. 2024;16:ep499.

Alexander E, White A, Varol A, Appel K, Lieneck C. Team- and problem-based learning in health services: a systematic literature review of recent initiatives in the United States. Educ Sci. 2024;14:515.

Ali M, Wahab IBA, Huri HZ, Yusoff MS. Personalised learning in higher education for health sciences: a scoping review protocol. Syst Rev. 2024;13:99.

Al-Zahrani AM. Enhancing postgraduate students' learning outcomes through flipped mobile-based microlearning. Res Learn Technol. 2024;32. https://doi.org/10.25304/rlt.v32.3110.

Atashinsadaf A, Ramezani-Badr F, Long T, Imanipour M, Amini K. Facilities, challenges, attitudes, and preferences of nursing students related to e-learning in the COVID-19 pandemic in Iranian context: a cross-sectional study. BMC Med Educ. 2024;24:50.

Boon İET. Self-regulated learning skills in instrument education: a qualitative study. Int J Educ Lit Stud. 2024;12:106–14.

Bose S, Bade JD, Naidu BRM, Roy P, Kandi V. Application of classroom assessment techniques in medical education: results from the community medicine teaching and learning experience. Cureus. 2024;16:e58930.

Chang WJ. Service-learning effectiveness and transformative learning among college students engaging in community services involving older adults with dementia. J Res Educ Sci. 2023;68:235–67.

Chang MC, Yu JH, Hsieh JG, Wei MH, Wang YW. Effectiveness of the refined health literacy course on improving the health literacy competencies of undergraduate nursing students: quantitative and qualitative perspectives. Med Educ Online. 2023;28:2173042.

Darmawansah D, Hwang GJ, Chen MRA, Liang JC. Trends and research foci of robotics-based STEM education: a systematic review from diverse angles based on the technology-based learning model. Int J STEM Educ. 2023;10:12.

Jebreen K, Radwan E, Kammoun-Rebai W, Alattar E, Radwan A, Safi W, Radwan W, Alajez M. Perceptions of undergraduate medical students on artificial intelligence in medicine: mixed-methods survey study from Palestine. BMC Med Educ. 2024;24:507.

Kerimbayev N, Umirzakova Z, Shadiev R, Jotsov V. A student-centered approach using modern technologies in distance learning: a systematic review of the literature. Smart Learn Environ. 2023;10:61.

Kilipiris F, Avdimiotis S, Christou E, Tragouda A, Konstantinidis I. Bloom's taxonomy student persona responses to blended learning methods employing the metaverse and flipped classroom tools. Educ Sci. 2024;14:418.

Leszczyński P, Gotlib J, Kopański Z, Wejnarski A, Świeżewski S, Gałązkowski R. Analysis of web-based learning methods in emergency medicine: randomized controlled trial. Arch Med Sci. 2018;14:687–94.

Medeiros GDS, Sousa ABV, Bezerra EF, Aragão LM, Rebouças HJ, Almeida EPO, De Pontes Filho RN, De Sousa MNA. Assessment of health education in the prevention of non-communicable chronic disease complications: systematic review. Rev Gest Soc Ambiental. 2024;18:e04904.

Páez DC, Flórez J, Gómez MT, García D, Arango-Paternina CM, Duperly J. Curricular and pedagogical approaches for physical activity prescription training: a mixed-methods study of the "exercise is medicine" workshops in Colombia. BMC Med Educ. 2024;24:79.

Rozhenkova V, Snow L, Sato BK, Lo SM, Buswell NT. Limited or complete? Teaching and learning conceptions and instructional environments fostered by STEM teaching versus research faculty. Int J STEM Educ. 2023;10:51.

Sany SBT, Behzhad F, Ferns G, Peyman N. Communication skills training for physicians improves health literacy and medical outcomes among patients with hypertension: a randomized controlled trial. BMC Health Serv Res. 2020;20:60.

Shrivastava SR, Shrivastava PS. Encouraging medical students to become self-directed learners through conduction of small-group learning sessions. J Nat Sci Med. 2021;4:90–1.

Tefera AS, Melaku EE, Urgie BM, Hassen EM, Tamene TD, Gebeyaw ED. Barriers to implementing problem-based learning at the school of medicine of Debre Berhan University, Ethiopia. BMC Med Educ. 2024;24:501.

Wankhar D, Kumar AP, Venugopal Vijayakumar A, Velan AB, Ravi P, Rudra B, Maheshkumar K. Effect of meditation, mindfulness-based stress reduction, and relaxation techniques as mind-body medicine practices to reduce blood pressure in cardiac patients: a systematic review and meta-analysis. Cureus. 2024;16:e58434.

Xiao S, Yuan J, Lan H, Li Q, Cheng Y, Cao K, Zeng X. Investigation of clinical medicine undergraduates' recognition of narrative medicine. BMC Med Educ. 2024;24:321.

Correction to: Students' Perspectives on the Pros and Cons of Current Instructional and Learning Methods

Amro Khalid Bin Abdulrahman and Hamad Saleh Alturki

Correction to:
Chapter 15 in: K. A. Bin Abdulrahman, H. Darami (eds.),
Essential Learning Skills for Health Professions Students,
https://doi.org/10.1007/978-981-96-5670-7_15

This title was recently published. The first author of Chapter 15 with affiliation and email address was published incorrectly and has been corrected with updated details.

The updated version of this chapter can be found at:
https://doi.org/10.1007/978-981-96-5670-7_15

K. A. Bin Abdulrahman, H. Darami (eds.), *Essential Learning Skills for Health Professions Students*, https://doi.org/10.1007/978-981-96-5670-7_16

MIX
Papier aus verantwortungsvollen Quellen
Paper from responsible sources
FSC® C105338

If you have any concerns about our products,
you can contact us on
ProductSafety@springernature.com

In case Publisher is established outside the EU,
the EU authorized representative is:
Springer Nature Customer Service Center GmbH
Europaplatz 3, 69115 Heidelberg, Germany

Printed by Libri Plureos GmbH
in Hamburg, Germany